The Hijacking of American Medicine
by Managed Care
The Perspective of a Practicing Physician

The Hijacking of American Medicine by Managed Care

The Perspective of a Practicing Physician

Arthur Gale MD

2004

The Hijacking of American Medicine by Managed Care

The Perspective of a Practicing Physician

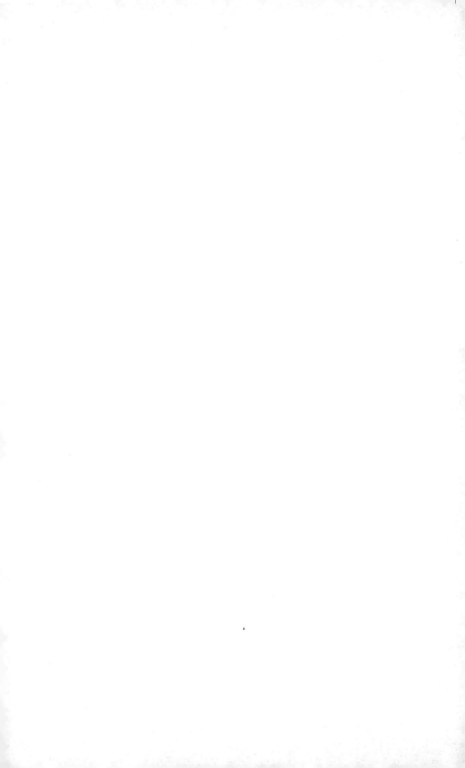

Table of Contents

Part One

The Courts Foster Managed Care

Part Two

Managed Care Escapes Regulation and Accountability

Part Three

Hospitals Change Their Mission to Meet Threat of Managed Care

Part Four

Managed Care is a Failure

Forward

A decade ago managed care appeared in my private office in the form of an HMO representative. He explained to me how the gatekeeper HMO worked. Doctors would be paid financial bonuses for ordering fewer tests and procedures and making fewer referrals to specialists. Patients were not to be informed about these perverse financial incentives.

I told the representative that I ordered tests and made referrals based on what I thought was necessary for my patients' welfare. I considered such financial incentives and their concealment from patients unethical. One word led to another and we parted acrimoniously. Since that time I have, with rare exception, not accepted HMO patients.

I could not understand how a health care system that employed such deceptive and dishonest practices could be imposed upon a free nation. I had been an attending physician on the internal medicine service of a respected teaching-community hospital for many years. I taught medical students and residents. I looked upon the academic medical center and the faculty as a role model for how physicians should practice medicine. I knew many academic physicians felt the same way I did about managed care. Why didn't their leadership speak out? Why didn't the government speak out? Why didn't the leadership of organized medicine speak out? Why didn't the public speak out?

There were other questions. How was managed care forced upon the American people without their approval? Who was behind the corporate managed care takeover of medicine? Why wouldn't or couldn't the public take legal action against managed care organizations when their deceptive practices led to patient harm. How were insurance companies able to force unfair one-sided contracts upon physicians? Why did hospitals become large horizontally and vertically integrated corporate conglomerates? Why has managed care's so-called free market economics model as applied to health care failed to control health care costs while the number of uninsured has increased?

I set out upon a quest to find answers to these and other questions about managed care. My quest was carried out over a 10-year period while I was engaged in active medical practice. I researched newspaper articles, books and journals, both medical and non-medical. I read judicial decisions. I experienced firsthand, as well as read about, the major role hospitals play in managed care. I discussed managed care with medical colleagues wherever I could - in my office, in hospital lunchrooms, in doctors' lounges and at medical meetings. No erudite academic journal, article or book can provide the real world knowledge of how managed care actually works better than can a practicing physician.

I found answers to the questions I raised. The reader may be as surprised as I was to discover that managed care was not just the creation of the health insurance industry that developed and marketed HMOs. Without the backing of the U.S. Supreme Court and Federal Trade Commission, as well as big business and academia, managed care could never have been imposed upon the American people without their approval.

Managed care ideology is based on three major assumptions. 1) Competition and the introduction of so-called free market economics into the health care delivery system will lower health care costs. 2) The fee-for-service method of paying doctors (and hospitals) is the prime culprit responsible for spiraling health care costs. 3) HMOs, through capitation, will change doctors' financial incentives and bring down health care costs. Leaders in government, business and academia bought this ideology. Many still hold these unproven assumptions as articles of faith.

Whatever ideological beliefs one holds, the facts are clear. Managed care hasn't worked. A decade ago, the country experienced double-digit annual health care inflation and there were 31 million uninsured Americans. Today, there is double-digit annual health care inflation and 42 million uninsured Americans. Presently the only players in managed care who profit from the system are the large managed care organizations and the hospital networks. The roles of these two oligopolies are discussed at length in this book. Large corporations, among the original and most zealous proponents of managed care, have seen their employee medical costs rise through the roof. They are beginning to have second thoughts about managed care.

I personally sympathize with the laudable goal of trying to lower health care costs. In addition to being a doctor, I am a small businessman. I am on the executive committee of an independent multi-specialty medical group that has about 60 employees. With low reimbursement rates from third party payers and spiraling malpractice premiums, it is difficult enough to meet a payroll, much less pay health insurance for our employees. Nevertheless, we have never purchased HMO plans for our employees or ourselves.

Before the country moves on to the next stage of health care reform, it is important that the public and physicians alike understand how and why managed care came about so that the same mistakes will not be repeated.

The essays in this short book were selected from a larger number of articles that appeared in the St. Louis Metropolitan Medical Society journal, *St. Louis Metropolitan Medicine*, and the Missouri State Medical Association journal, *Missouri Medicine*. The articles were written primarily for my physician colleagues, but I believe that the general public also will find these essays informative.

Although I have researched topics carefully, the essays are essentially opinion pieces. They contain occasional references, but not footnotes. They are presented according to subject matter rather than in chronological order.

I wish to thank the American Medical Association where I have served as an alternate delegate and delegate for a number of years, as well as the St. Louis Metropolitan Medical Society and the Missouri State Medical Association for their patience and forbearance in allowing me to express my strong, and sometimes unconventional, views on managed care. The views expressed in this book are mine and do not represent the official policies of any of these organizations.

I also wish to thank my medical colleagues who, by their support and encouragement, have kept me writing all these years. I wish most of all to thank my wife, Marilyn, who against all odds enabled me to write clear and I hope comprehensible prose.

Arthur H. Gale, M.D.
2003

Part One

The Courts Foster Managed Care

U.S. Supreme Court and Federal Trade Commission Determine Medicine is Not a Profession

Decision Affects Patient Care
Missouri Medicine
July 1997

When did physicians cease being professionals and become mere purveyors of commerce? When did physicians become providers and patients become customers? Who is responsible for physicians' no longer being advocates for their patients' health, while working under the perverse financial incentives of capitation which reward them for withholding care?

Most persons would probably answer that these changes in the practice of medicine were brought about gradually over the past decade or so by business and insurance interests in order to lower costs. That answer is not correct. The prime movers for these changes were the U.S. Supreme Court and the Federal Trade Commission. The year in which these changes began was 1975.

In 1975, Lewis and Ruth Goldfarb contracted to buy a home. This required employing an attorney to conduct a title examination. All of the lawyers whom they contacted charged a similar fee. The Goldfarbs filed suit contending that the Virginia State Bar and local bar association conspired to restrain interstate commerce through the use of fixed fees. The case went all the way to the U.S. Supreme Court. The Court ruled in favor of the Goldfarbs.

The Goldfarb suit did not directly involve any physician or physician organizations. Yet it was to become a landmark decision with devastating effects on the medical profession.

The court ruled that henceforth the learned professions, law and medicine were to be treated like any other commercial activity and were not exempt from antitrust. All of the changes in the practice of medicine over the past two decades can be traced to that one decision. Most doctors have never heard of it.

As pointed out by Kuttner (*New England Journal of Medicine*, Jan. 30, 1997), the Court's position on the medical profession was best summarized in an amicus brief for the plaintiffs filed by a prominent antitrust law professor. The brief included the following statement, "The success of the medical profession in controlling the economic environment of physicians from the 1930s to the 1980s ... was arguably the most successful restraint of trade ever perpetrated by private interests against American consumers."

Now, more than two decades after the Goldfarb decision, and with managed care the dominant form of health care delivery, some of the original supporters of the Goldfarb decision are having misgivings. Because of the commercialization of the medical marketplace by the giant for-profit HMOs, the trust, which has traditionally existed between patient and doctor, has eroded. This trust has been replaced by the credo of the marketplace—"caveat emptor" or buyer beware.

The naive assumption by the Supreme Court that the profession of medicine could be treated like any other commercial activity is belied by the rising tide of public outrage against the abuses of managed care.

The recent passage of the managed care bill, HB 335, by the Missouri legislature is just one of many pieces of legislation introduced in the U.S. over the past several years attempting to regulate these abuses.

The Goldfarb decision was wrong because it transferred control of patient care from the medical profession with its code of ethics dating back to the Hippocratic Oath, to the FTC and, to a lesser degree, the Department of Justice, Antitrust Division.

An FTC attorney (*New England Journal of Medicine*, Oct. 3, 1985) wrote, "The FTC's responsibility is to preserve and foster competitive opportunities and consumer choice in the marketplace ..." Most physicians, I believe, would not quarrel with that definition of antitrust. Physicians are not afraid of competition based on cost and quality.

There are, however, significant problems with physicians' ability to comply with the FTC goals. First, under managed care, "competitive opportunities" exist only for insurance companies competing for the business of employers, not physicians competing for the business of consumers. Second, there is virtually no "consumer choice." The consumer (employee) is auctioned off once a year like a commodity to the HMO tendering the lowest bid to the employer. Third, the medical "marketplace" is unnatural because of third party payers; it is not a marketplace of individual consumers freely making choice based on quality and cost, as intended by the FTC statement.

In 1979, the FTC filed a successful antitrust suit against the AMA over the AMA's "anti competitive ethical restrictions" on free choice of physician, compensation on a non fee-for-service basis, the corporate practice of medicine and truthful advertising. The term "non fee-for-service" is a euphemism for capitation. Three years later, the FTC issued a restraining order preventing the AMA Council on Ethical and Judicial Affairs from even issuing a non-binding opinion on the ethics of capitation which involve withholds and bonuses. And more recently the FTC has issued rules preventing physicians from forming networks unless the doctors assume financial risk for patient care.

The FTC brooks no dissent on the ethics of capitation, withholds, bonuses, physicians at financial risk, and the harm to patients, which these practices may cause. The FTC has effectively silenced its critics in organized medicine by threatening the AMA with a lawsuit if it spoke out against the ethics of capitation. The FTC dismissed the AMA's ethical concerns about capitation as just a ploy to preserve the economic interests of its members.

Thus we are witness to the FTC's transformation from a regulatory agency charged with enforcing free and open competition to becoming a laboratory for social engineering. The FTC has decided on its own to impose a revolutionary and untried system of capitation on the American people without their prior informed consent.

The FTC has one all-consuming goal—to lower health care costs. As such, the agency's position is essentially amoral. It chooses to ignore the possibility that this new system of capitation carries the potential of harming patients. It ignores the possibility that financial incentives in the form of withholds and bonuses can affect patient care by denying appropriate tests, procedures, and physician referrals.

The justices who wrote the majority decision in the Goldfarb case and the Congressmen who enacted the Sherman Antitrust Act of 1890, as well as those persons in the Woodrow Wilson administration who created the

FTC, probably never heard of capitation or envisioned the role of the FTC in promoting it.

Now we are beginning to see capitation under attack by the public, the media, ethicists, the legal profession, and the courts. The public is beginning to recognize the fallout from capitation as practiced by managed care companies—poor patient care, denial of benefits, and lack of accountability.

The managed care industry has foolishly and unsuccessfully used gag rules in an attempt to conceal capitation and its perverse financial incentives from the public. By imposing gag rules on doctors, managed care virtually admits it is doing something wrong—something that it doesn't want the public to know about.

The FTC has provided no antitrust remedy for the abuses against consumers by managed care companies. And under ERISA, the law, which covers 50 percent to 60 percent of employed persons in the U.S., injured parties have no right to redress their grievances against managed care companies through the courts.

The FTC cannot dismiss public concern over the ethics of capitation as it has physician concern by threatening a lawsuit against the AMA. An aroused public opinion is forcing the FTC and its supporters to reassess its position on capitation and doctors assuming financial risk.

Administrative agencies like the FTC are supposed to be a part of the executive branch of government administering laws passed by Congress. In fact they often act like a fourth branch of government wielding enormous power, making new rules which differ significantly from the intent of the original laws passed by Congress.

Administrative agencies are often unaccountable until they step out of line too far and Congress has to pass additional laws to rein them in. This actually happened in the last Congress when the threat of legislation (Hyde) forced the FTC to change its policy on physician-sponsored networks.

Ultimately it is the public who will render the final judgment on our present system of health care delivery spawned by the Goldfarb decision as interpreted and implemented by the FTC. In our system of government it is the people who are the final source of authority. If the public becomes disenchanted with the major features of managed care—capitation, perverse financial incentives, gag rules, and lack of consumer choice and protection, no branch of government can prevent its collapse.

Two U.S. Supreme Court Decisions Give Control of Medical Ethics to the FTC

Public's Trust in Health Care Plummets
Missouri Medicine
September 1997

American medicine faces an ethical crisis. In the past two decades, two U.S. Supreme Court decisions have changed medical ethics and the way physicians practice more radically than any other event since Hippocrates wrote his famous oath 2,400 years ago. Despite their importance, almost none of the nation's 700,000 physicians have even heard of these landmark decisions.

The first decision was the Goldfarb case in 1975. (*Missouri Medicine*, July 1997.) In that case the Court ruled that medicine was no longer a learned profession. The practice of medicine was to be considered no differently from any other commercial activity and was henceforth subject to antitrust regulations, which were to be administered mainly by the Federal Trade Commission.

The second Supreme Court case, FTC vs. the American Medical Association concluded in 1980. In this decision the FTC found that ethical standards issued by the AMA were in violation of the Federal Trade Commission. By winning this case, the FTC gained control over the AMA's Council on Ethical and Judicial Affairs, which is the AMA body that issues ethical opinions. By obtaining veto power over CEJA opinions, the FTC effectively neutralized AMA ethical opposition to HMOs. The FTC-sponsored managed care revolution could then proceed smoothly and rapidly.

Shortly after the Goldfarb decision, the FTC wasted no time in exercising its newfound control over organized medicine. It filed an antitrust suit against the AMA. The antitrust suit attacked the heart of the AMA—its code of ethics. The 1975 AMA code of ethics with its preamble is printed in Table 1. Even today it is difficult to find fault with any of its provisions.

The FTC basically attacked sections five and six. The FTC interpreted section five as prohibiting advertising and fee disclosure, and section six as prohibiting doctors from being employed on a contract basis (such as by an HMO).

Despite a valiant legal defense by the AMA, the courts unfortunately agreed with the FTC. The AMA lost in the lower courts. It lost in the Second Circuit Court of Appeals in a two-to-one decision. The U.S. Supreme Court in an equally divided 4-4 vote affirmed without comment the Federal Appeals Court decision. Justice Harry Blackmon recused himself because he had once represented the Mayo Clinic. Thus at both the Federal Appeals level and the Supreme Court level the AMA lost by just one vote.

The importance of these two decisions cannot be overestimated. The courts have essentially given the FTC the authority to ban any AMA ethical criticism of new forms of health care delivery such as HMOs. In addition the AMA has to write its code of ethics in such a way so that it is in compliance with the rules set by the FTC. The FTC monitors every recommendation and every policy issued by the CEJA.

The foremost example of the FTC's power over the AMA is an FTC order prohibiting CEJA from issuing restrictive ethical guidelines in the area of HMO financial incentives. Financial incentives are monetary bonuses paid to physicians for not ordering tests and procedures on patients and for not referring patients to specialists or to the hospital. It is obvious that financial incentives pit the interests of physicians against the interests of patients. Financial incentives are the heart of managed care. They are the fundamental means by which managed care achieves its savings. Until doctors were placed at financial risk over the past several years, HMOs did not lower medical costs. Therefore, an order restricting criticism of financial incentives is essentially an order restricting criticism of managed care. If CEJA went ahead anyway and criticized financial incentives in violation of the FTC order, its members and possibly the leadership of the AMA could be sent to jail.

AMA attorneys stated in court that the FTC's restraining order against CEJA violated the AMA's First Amendment freedom of speech rights. Two Federal Appeals Courts judges in an unusual line of reasoning disagreed. They said that freedom of speech can be limited as when, for example, two competitors meet and discuss price fixing. But a CEJA advisory opinion on the ethics of financial incentives is hardly a conspiracy to fix prices and restrain trade. CEJA does possess moral authority, but it has no legal authority to compel doctors to do anything.

Of all people, the Federal Appeals Court and the U.S. Supreme Court should know that criticizing the government or a policy of the government is not a crime. The Supreme Court not too long ago rendered an opinion that under the First Amendment that it's okay to burn the

American flag. But in another opinion the Supreme Court can turn around and decide that it's not okay for the AMA to advise its members on the ethics of HMO financial incentives.

Where is the consistency?

By taking over control of its ethical standards, the FTC has essentially made the medical profession a vassal of the state. History teaches us that when medical ethics are controlled by the whims of the state and not by a higher professional and moral code great harm to human beings can occur. For example after World War II, at the Nuremberg Doctor's Trial, Allied prosecutors tried German physicians who had committed atrocities in the name of experimental medicine and the advancement of science (*Journal of the American Medical Association*, Nov. 27, 1996). These doctors' actions were condoned and supported by the state. When the state takes control of medical ethics, the Hippocratic Oath, the AMA Code of Ethics, and all other codes of medical ethics become meaningless scraps of paper.

Judge Mansfield of the 2nd Federal Circuit Court of Appeals cites the pretrial prejudicial statements by the then director of the FTC, Michael Pertschuk. These statements illustrate the cynical opinion of the medical profession held by the movers and the shakers at the FTC. They also give insight into the goals of the FTC.

Pertschuk states, "While it would probably be excessive to say that the fox (the medical profession) is guarding the chicken coop, it is undeniable that a great many critical judgments in this field are being made by people with a direct economic stake in particular outcomes ... ."

Thus any criticism of HMO financial incentives on ethical grounds is dismissed by the FTC as a rationalization for protecting doctors' pocketbooks. This statement also justifies the FTC's lofty vision of its "mission" as elitist social engineers whose goal is to restructure American health care to better serve the needs of consumers.

But the FTC neglected to ask the American public its opinion of HMOs, which employ financial incentives. As a result it should come as no surprise that the public is not very happy with the results of the FTC's social engineering. Evidence is mounting that under managed care, consumers are losing their trust in health care.

I discussed these matters with an FTC antitrust attorney at a recent medical meeting.

I pointed out that:

1. The media across the nation bashes managed care on a fairly regular basis.
2. Independent public opinion polls ranked managed care very low--just above the tobacco industry in one survey.
3. At a Missouri legislative committee hearing in 1996, more than 150 persons gave 2,500 pages of testimony against managed care companies in attempting to get a bill passed which would regulate the excesses of managed care.
4. The legal system and the courts are successfully attacking and destroying the credibility of financial incentives.

I then asked the antitrust attorney if the FTC was satisfied with the results of its reengineering of the American health care system. He did not dispute the points that I had brought up, but his answer, to say the least, was disappointing. His response was that, "the market was evolving."

This is a standard bureaucratic response. If plans don't

work out as expected, take no responsibility and show no remorse.

In downtown St. Louis stands a stately pre-Civil War courthouse. Nestled among modern high-rises the Old Courthouse, as it is affectionately called, seems strangely out of place. But the Old Courthouse is more than a nostalgic reminder of a bygone period. It stands as a reminder—actually a monument to the fallibility of the U.S. Supreme Court. For in this courthouse, the infamous Dred Scott case took place—a case in which the Supreme Court ultimately declared that a human being was property.

There have been many bad decisions by the Supreme Court before and since Dred Scott. The Dred Scott case was eventually reversed. Most of the other bad Supreme Court decisions, which are not high profile such as Goldfarb and FTC vs. AMA, will likely remain on the books forever.

But there is in our democratic society a court even higher than the Supreme Court. It is called the court of public opinion. The public, not the FTC and not the courts, will render the final opinion on the ethics of the U.S. health care system of the future. The public will make a choice either of FTC-sponsored ethics characterized by financial incentives, physician guile, and patient mistrust; or the public will chose a health care system based upon more than 2,000 years of professional ethics, characterized by openness and honesty where physicians practice as patient advocates.

❧

Table 1 — AMA Principles of Ethics, 1975

1. PRINCIPLES OF MEDICAL ETHICS
PREAMBLE

These principles are intended to aid physicians individually and collectively in maintaining a high level of ethical conduct. They are not laws but standards by which a physician may determine the propriety of his conduct in his relationship with patients, with colleagues, with members of allied professions, and with the public.

SECTION 1: The principle objective of the medical profession is to render service to humanity with full respect for the dignity of man. Physicians should merit the confidence of patients entrusted to their care, rendering to each a full measure of service and devotion.

SECTION 2: Physicians should strive continually to improve medical knowledge and skill, and should make available to their patients and colleagues the benefits of their professional attainments.

SECTION 3: A physician should practice a method of healing founded on a scientific basis; and he should not voluntarily associate professionally with anyone who violates this principle.

SECTION 4: The medical profession should safeguard the public and itself against physicians deficient in moral character or professional competence. Physicians should observe all laws, uphold the dignity and honor of the profession and accept its self-imposed disciplines. They should expose, without hesitation, illegal or unethical conduct of fellow members of the profession.

SECTION 5: A physician may choose whom he will serve. In an emergency, however, he should render service to the best of his ability. Having undertaken the care of a patient, he may not neglect him; and unless he has been discharged he may discontinue his services only after giving adequate notice. He should not solicit patients.

SECTION 6: A physician should not dispose of his services under terms or conditions which tend to interfere with or impair the free and complete exercise of his medical judgment and skill or tend to cause a deterioration of the quality of medical care.

SECTION 7: In the practice of medicine, a physician should limit the source of his professional income to medical services actually rendered by him, or under his supervision, to his patients. His fee should be commensurate with the services rendered and the patient's ability to pay. He should neither pay nor receive a commission for referral of patients. Drugs, remedies or appliances may be dispensed or supplied by the physician provided it is in the best interests of the patients.

SECTION 8: A physician should seek consultation upon request; in doubtful or difficult cases; or whenever it appears that the quality of medical service may be enhanced thereby.

SECTION 9: A physician may not reveal the confidences entrusted to him in the course of medical attendance, or the deficiencies he may observe in the character of patients, unless he is required to do so by law or unless it becomes necessary in order to protect the welfare of the individual or of the community.

SECTION 10: The honored ideals of the medical profession imply that the responsibilities of the physician extend not only to the individual, but also to society where these responsibilities deserved his interest and participation in activities which have the purpose of improving both the health and the well being of the individual and the community.

1982 Supreme Court Decision Destroys Fee-For-Service

Fosters HMOs with Financial Incentives

Missouri Medicine
December 1997

In 1982, the U.S. Supreme Court in a four-to-three decision ruled that the Maricopa and Pima County medical societies in Arizona could not form a medical foundation, which set maximum (not minimum) fees.

By setting up a medical foundation, the Maricopa County medical society wanted in the Court's words, "to provide the community with a competitive alternative to existing health insurance plans." The doctors wanted to preserve fee-for-service medicine. Health insurance companies were willing to negotiate with the foundation because under such a system they could better predict their costs.

The goals of the Maricopa County doctors were laudable. How many times have physicians heard from colleagues and the public that doctors have brought on their own problems because of exorbitant fees charged by some physicians. The Maricopa County doctors simply wanted to eliminate that problem. Competition would be preserved because physicians would still be able to set fees as low as they wished.

The Court, however, ruled that any price fixing including the setting of maximum fees was a per se violation of the Sherman Antitrust Act. The term per se essentially means the literal interpretation of any law. In the case of the Sherman Act, a per se interpretation would mean that any and all forms of price fixing are prohibited.

The defendants and the minority of the Court (Powell, Rehnquist and Chief Justice Burger) believed that the role of reason not the per se rule should apply. Justice Louis Brandeis provided the classic definition of the rule of reason. Boiled down to its basics, it means in antitrust cases that if the intent and outcome of price fixing promotes competition, it is legal. Rule of reason also allows facts unique to the particular case to be brought before the court. The minority opinion cited precedents where price fixing was ruled legal according to the rule of reason.

If the views of the minority had prevailed, if one vote of the Supreme Court had been changed, the takeover of American medicine by HMOs and managed care companies might never have occurred. A significant role for fee-for-service medicine might have been preserved.

Justice Powell, writing the dissenting opinion made some telling comments and issued some stern warnings, "Medical services differ from the typical service or commercial product at issue in an antitrust case. The services of physicians ... rarely can be compared by the recipient. A person requiring medical service or advice has no ready way of comparing physicians or shopping for quality medical service at a lesser price. Primarily for this reason, the foundations ... perform a function that neither physicians nor prospective patients can perform individually ... We thus have a case in which we derive little guidance from the conventional 'perfect market' analysis of antitrust law. I would give greater weight than the (majority) Court to the uniqueness of medical services, and certainly would not invalidate on a per se basis a plan that may in fact perform a uniquely useful service ... It is unwise for the Court, in a case as novel and important as this one, to make a final judgment in the absence of a complete record."

In essence, the dissenting judges warned the Court majority that since medical care was unique and unlike the manufacturing and marketing of commercial products, their ruling could have unintended harmful consequences. Now 25 years later, with managed care firmly entrenched, events are bearing out their well-founded concerns.

There is another legacy of the Maricopa decision, which has had an even more destructive impact on health care and the doctor-patient relationship than just the elimination of fee-for-service.

The Court advocated a revolutionary and untried method of health care deliver—HMOs, capitation, and physicians, not insurance companies, assuming financial risk when caring for patients.

The Court's opinion state, "Most health insurance plans are of the fee-for-service type. Under the typical insurance plan, the insurer agrees with the insured to reimburse the insured for 'usual, customary, and reasonable' medical charges. The third party insurer, and the insured to the extent of any excess charges, bears the economic risk that the insured will require medical treatment. An alternative to the fee-for-service type of insurance plan is illustrated by health maintenance organizations authorized under the Health Maintenance Organization Act of 1970 ... Under this form of prepaid health plan, the consumer pays a fixed periodic fee to a functionally integrated group of doctors in exchange for the group's agreement to provide any medical treatment that the subscriber might need. *The economic risk is thus borne by the doctors."* (Italics mine.)

To my knowledge this is the first time that the Supreme Court ever applied the concept of physicians assuming economic risk to health care. The legal foundation upon which the Federal Trade Commission manages health care is based primarily upon this one sentence. Unfortunately, most of the ethical problems faced by managed care today can also be attributed to this one sentence.

The Court's pronouncement on "alternative to the fee-for-service type of insurance plan" reflects its political and social agenda in fostering HMOs, capitation, financial incentives, and physicians assuming financial risk. It illustrates the Court's self-appointed role as social engineer imposing a health care delivery system upon the American people without their prior approval. It also illustrates the Court's limited knowledge of the success of HMOs in reducing costs up until 1982 when the Maricopa decision was rendered. Had the Court taken the position of the dissenting justices and followed the rule of reason they might have learned some interesting facts.

The Health Maintenance Organization Act of 1973 was enacted under the Nixon administration. Nixon hailed from California. His advisors cited the Kaiser Permanente physician-sponsored HMO as a cost-cutting paradigm for future health care delivery. However, numerous studies in the 1970s and 1980s failed to show that HMOs reduced costs. Doctors practicing in group-model HMOs like Kaiser reduced hospitalization days by up to 40 percent. But outpatient utilization increased and ultimate cost savings were insignificant. The conclusion to be drawn from the studies of the '70s and '80s was that when doctors practiced according to their best medical judgment there were no significant cost differences between fee-for-service and HMOs.

This conclusion is as true today as it was in the 1970s and 1980s. Two recent studies tracking medical costs (*Health Affairs*, Fall 1996 and July, August 1997) show that cost reductions in recent years under fee-for-service just about matched the drop in costs under HMOs. The most likely reason for this surprising finding is that most physicians, no matter under what plan they practice, admit fewer patients to the hospital and for shorter stays than they did in past years. Yet managed care dogma states unequivocally that fee-for-service is the culprit responsible for high medical costs despite the lack of evidence to support this notion.

In Maricopa, the Court's comments on risk assumption by doctors applied primarily to staff model HMOs with which the justices were familiar. Staff model HMOs like Kaiser dominated the market in 1982. The Court declared "the consumer pays a fixed periodic fee to a functionally integrated group of doctors ... The economic risk is thus borne by the doctors."

The FTC and commercial HMOs have taken this restrictive definition of risk out of context and expanded it. Under present day managed care, risk pools are set up which include doctors who are not functionally integrated. The Department of Health and Human Services has taken the concept of risk even further in Medicare HMOs. The individual doctor is at financial risk for his panel of patients. If, through no fault of his own, he encounters seriously ill patients whom he must admit to the hospital, he can be personally liable for tens of thousands of dollars.

When doctors work under financial risk they have a strong temptation to withhold necessary care, which can result in patient harm. It is no wonder then that the three largest not-for-profit HMOs, including Kaiser, have joined the consumers in backing sweeping regulations to control the abuses of managed care which include financial incentives (*New York Times*, Sept. 25, 1997). One of the standards being sought by Kaiser and other non-profit HMOs is, "Health plans should not pay doctors in any way that directly encourages them to limit medically necessary care." Ironically, this swipe at financial incentives is a direct repudiation of the goals of the Supreme Court (and FTC) by the very organizations, which served as the model for the Maricopa decision.

If the Supreme Court were to assess today, the managed care revolution which it helped initiate, its members might be shocked. They might be shocked at how their well-intentioned decisions played a decisive role in the breakdown in the bond of trust between doctor and patient. They might be shocked at how the FTC, HHS, and commercial insurers have expanded and distorted their original concept of risk and installed financial incentives, which pervade almost every aspect of the doctor-patient relationship. They might be shocked by the actions of an angry public attempting to enact 2,000 pieces of legislation in order to regulate the managed care revolution which they helped spawn. They might be shocked that the very HMOs, which served as, the model for their opinion in Maricopa are asking for "legally enforceable national standards" to restore the public's confidence in managed care.

The Supreme Court might well be shocked by these events but the justices should not be surprised. The managed care revolution for which their opinions helped pave the way has something in common with the failed revolutions which occurred earlier this century in the Soviet Union, Italy and Germany. All of these revolutions placed the goals of society—"the common good"—above the rights of the individual. In the case of managed care, the benefit to society of reducing medical costs is deemed a goal more worthy than the health of an individual who may require expensive care. The current backlash against managed care is the public's way of telling the Court and the proponents of managed care in government and the private sector that they will not accept that goal. They are telling the social engineers of the last three decades loudly and clearly that this is not the American way.

U.S. Supreme Court Validates HMO Financial Incentives and Further Undermines Professionalism in the Practice of Medicine

Missouri Medicine
October 2000

Recently the U.S. Supreme Court in a unanimous decision validated physician financial incentives, even if the incentives contribute to harming a patient. As stated in Justice Souter's opinion, "The question in this case is whether treatment decisions made by a health maintenance organization, acting through its physician employees, are fiduciary acts within the meaning of the Employee Retirement Income Security Act of 1974. We hold that they are not." The Supreme Court reversed the Federal Appeals Court's decision, which had come to precisely the opposite conclusion.

The case of Herdich vs. Peagram was about a patient with abdominal pain and a pelvic mass who had to wait eight days for a pelvic ultrasound to be performed at a facility used by her physician's HMO. During this period of time the patient's appendix ruptured and she developed peritonitis. She could have had the ultrasound performed in a more timely fashion at a nearby hospital ... Herdrich successfully sued her physician for malpractice.

Herdrich believed that she could also sue the HMO under a provision of ERISA. She contended that HMO financial incentives to withhold care constituted a breach of fiduciary duty to the patient.

What is a fiduciary's duty in general and what is a fiduciary's to an employee-patient under ERISA? The Supreme Court's answer to these two questions has tremendous significance for the doctor-patient relationship.

The Court's opinion says that under ERISA fiduciaries shall discharge their duties with respect to a plan "solely in the interests of the participants and beneficiaries." The opinion goes on: "Responsibilities under ERISA have the familiar ring of their source as the common law of trusts. The common law charges fiduciaries with a duty of loyalty to guarantee beneficiary's interests ... and must exclude all selfish interest and all considerations of the interests of third persons. A trustee is held to something stricter than the market place ..." So far this definition of a fiduciary's duty sounds pretty much like a doctor's relationship to a patient under the Hippocratic Oath.

But then Souter backs off and says that the common law definition of fiduciary duty does not apply to the doctor-patient relationship. It applies only to a trustee's relationship to a trust. It has to do with guardianship of money such as is held in a pension or retirement plan. The Court's opinion then proceeds to propound a long and involved argument as to why the doctor's role as guardian of a patient's health under ERISA is of a lower order than a trustee's guardianship of a person's financial wealth.

Under ERISA the fiduciary duty of a doctor to a patient is not as strict as that of a trustee to a pension plan because the physician's decisions are "mixed" and contain elements not only of diagnosis and treatment but "eligibility" of patients for plan benefits.

The Court cites the Health Maintenance Organization Act passed by Congress in 1973 under the Nixon administration as the source of this new definition of the doctor-patient relationship. The Court states that, under the HMO Act Congress intended that physicians act not only on behalf of patients but also on behalf of the company, which contracted with the HMO to administer the plan. The company must weigh the interests of the for-profit company against the needs of the patient. Thus the role of the doctor is "mixed" and, according to the Court of a lower order than that of a true fiduciary.

This type of hair-splitting reasoning just doesn't make sense in the real world. Most physicians try to treat all patients the same—according to their best medical judgment. It doesn't make any difference whether a patient is covered under ERISA, under Medicare, under individually owned insurance, or even whether the patient has no insurance.

The Supreme Court's definition of a physician's duty under ERISA is artificial and contrary to the Hippocratic Oath. Furthermore it probably does not represent the intention of Congress in 1973 when the HMO Act was passed. In 1973 there were virtually no gatekeeper HMOs and no examples of financial incentives to withhold or delay care.

There were staff model HMOs like Kaiser, which assumed financial risk. These staff model HMOs held promise for reducing health care costs. However, in the 1970s and 1980s there were numerous studies that showed that staff model HMOs achieved no cost savings compared to fee-for-service when physicians practiced according to their best medical judgment.

For the Court to say that Congress intended that physicians treat patients insured under ERISA HMO plans according to a different and lesser standard than other patients (and to a different standard from a trustee in charge of a person's financial assets) is simply inconsistent with the facts. Many of these Congressmen would likely be appalled at the Court's interpretation of the law. They did not foresee physicians becoming "company doctors" rather than independent professionals under either the Federal HMO Act or ERISA.

The Supreme Court's interpretation of Herdrich vs. Peagram is in keeping with its previous decisions commercializing the practice of medicine. In the 1975 decision Goldfarb (*Missouri Medicine*, July 1997), the Supreme Court declared that medicine (and law) were no longer learned professions exempt from antitrust law but "ordinary purveyors of commerce." This decision essentially handed over control of medical ethics to the Federal trade Commission. In the 1980 decision AMA vs. FTC (*Missouri Medicine*, September 1997), the Supreme Court backed the FTC's demand that the AMA remove two Principles from its Principles of Medical Ethics. One of these Principles is virtually a mirror image of the Hippocratic Oath. In Herdrich vs. Peagram, the Supreme Court in effect finalizes the removal of professional standards from the practice of medicine.

The response of various interest groups to this decision is worth noting. The HMO industry, as expected, hailed the decision as validating their methods of controlling costs. The trial lawyers are not dismayed by the decision, however. They say they are not challenging the practices that managed care uses to save money. They are challenging their misrepresentations and failure to make truthful disclosures about those practices, just as they did in their class action victories over big tobacco. The AMA supports that part of the decision which states that ERISA and the federal courts are not the place to seek redress of grievances against HMOs. The decision affirms AMA policy that a strong federal patient protection bill is needed so that patients can seek legal remedies in state courts.

It is difficult to comprehend the Supreme Court's conclusion that a trustee's guardianship of a person's wealth is more important than a physician's guardianship of a person's health. Reading the Supreme Court decision reminded me of a famous radio routine by the comedian Jack Benny. In the skit a robber holds up Benny at gunpoint.

Robber: "Your money or your life."

Benny: Silence.

Audience: Laughter.

Robber (after several minutes and by now exasperated): "Make up your mind, your money or your life!"

Benny: "I'm thinking. I'm thinking."

Audience: More laughter.

Although the audience laughter after Benny's words "I'm thinking" is reputed to have been the longest in radio history, the Supreme Court justices would fail to see the humor because in Herdrich vs. Peagram, they decided that your money *is* more important than your life. Most Americans, especially those with health problems would not agree with the Supreme Court that wealth is more important than health. They don't want their physicians to have divided or "mixed" loyalty, part to the HMO and employer, and part to them. That is why 80 percent of the public supports a strong patient bill of rights to make HMOs accountable when their decisions harm them.

Passage of a strong patient bill of rights would neutralize the three Supreme Court decisions that have undermined professionalism in the practice of medicine. By making HMOs accountable, physicians could again practice independently and according to the tenets of the Hippocratic Oath.

AMA Restores Hippocratic Oath to Medical Ethics

Missouri Medicine
December 2001

The major reason for the founding of the AMA in 1847 was the medical profession's need to establish a code of ethical standards. In 1847 crass commercialism was pervasive in health care. Diploma mills flourished. Physicians and non-physicians alike sold quack medicines and cures. The public began to lose trust and confidence in the medical profession. As a means of restoring public confidence the newly formed AMA established a code of medical ethics.

The restoration of public trust by establishing a code of ethical standards is as important and valid today as it was in 1847 because of the commercialism that characterizes our current health care delivery system.

At the Annual 2001 meeting, the AMA House of Delegates adopted a new revision of the Principles of Medical Ethics. This is only the fourth time in the AMA's 154-year history that the Principles have been changed. The revision contains a new Section VIII that resulted from a Missouri resolution introduced at the A-1998 AMA meeting.

Section VIII states, "A physician shall, while caring for the patient, regard responsibility to the patient as paramount." This short and simple statement reasserts the physician's traditional role as patient advocate. This role has been absent from the previous Principles for over two decades. In order to understand just how important the new Section VIII is, a brief historical background is in order.

Most physicians and the public are unaware that the last revision of the Principles in 1980 was not initiated by the AMA but was mandated by the government. The AMA fought the government's takeover of medical ethics in two bitterly contested court cases. The AMA lost both cases.

In the first case, Goldfarb (1975) (*Missouri Medicine*, July 1997), the U.S. Supreme Court decided that the professions of law and medicine were no longer to be considered learned professions exempt from antitrust laws. They were to be considered in the words of the Court "ordinary purveyors of commerce" and under the control of the Federal Trade Commission and the Department of Justice. This landmark decision, hardly known to either physicians or the general public, constitutes the legal authority for the commercialization and the loss of ethical standards in the delivery of health care that has occurred over the past two decades. The Supreme Court's intent in placing the practice of medicine under the control of the FTC was to lower health care costs through free market competition.

The ink was hardly dry on the Goldfarb decision when the FTC sued the AMA specifically over its Principles of Medical Ethics (*Missouri Medicine*, September 1997). In a two-to-one decision in favor of the FTC, the U.S. Second Circuit Court of Appeals compelled the AMA to remove Sections 5 and 6 from the 1975 Principles. The U.S. Supreme Court in a split four-to-four decision refused to hear the case. Section 5 prohibited doctors from advertising. Section 6 was of far greater importance and constitutes the heart of medical ethics-patient advocacy.

Section 6 of the 1975 Principles is printed in the sidebar. It is virtually a mirror image of the Hippocratic Oath, which is also contained in the sidebar. The Hippocratic Oath and Section 6 both declare that physicians, in practicing medicine, should use their "best medical judgment and avoid what is deleterious" or harmful to the patient.

The FTC interpreted the initial clause of Section 6 "A physician should not dispose of his services under terms or conditions which tend to interfere with or impair the free and complete exercise of his medical judgment" as restraint of trade. The FTC concluded that the clause implied that physicians should not join HMOs for ethical reasons. By forcing the removal of Section 6 from the 1975 AMA Principles the FTC has implicitly endorsed the position that it's OK for physicians to not use their best medical judgment and not avoid what is harmful to patients. This position is indefensible and would not be acceptable to the majority of the American people if they were aware of it.

As a result of the Goldfarb and AMA vs. FTC decisions a historical precedent with enormous and frightening consequences has been established wherein two branches of our federal government, the Supreme Court and the FTC, have told doctors that they can no longer practice medicine according to the Hippocratic Oath. These two judicial decisions have essentially handed over control of medical ethics from physicians to the FTC.

It is not surprising then that the initial reaction of physicians to the administrative law judge's conclusions in the 1975 FTC vs. AMA suit was "outrage that non-physicians would presume to be experts in establishing ethical standards for the medical profession."

The removal of Section VI from the 1975 Principles is

not just of academic interest. To this very day AMA vs. FTC prohibits the AMA from advising any physician "on the ethical propriety" of any contract that the physician might enter into. It also prohibits the AMA Council on Ethical and Judicial Affairs from issuing restrictive guidelines in the area of HMO financial incentives. Financial incentives can violate the Hippocratic Oath because they pit the financial interests of the physician against the medical needs of the patient.

The physician reaction of "outrage" in 1975 to the government's takeover of medical ethics was certainly appropriate, given the historical record of the 20th century. Under National Socialism the German medical profession, once the world's finest, descended to unimaginable depths by embracing a state-sponsored ideology. If German doctors had followed the Hippocratic dictum of using their best medical judgment and avoiding what is detrimental to the patient, they would not have perpetrated horrible atrocities in their experiments involving human subjects. Likewise, had Soviet psychiatrists followed the Hippocratic dictum of not harming patients instead of the then current communist ideology, they would not have incarcerated political dissidents in psychiatric hospitals. These examples may sound extreme but they teach us how important it is for the medical profession to remain free to adhere to its own fundamental code of ethics dating back 2,500 years. A government takeover of medical ethics for any ideology, even one that espouses free market economics, is suspect. The FTC and Supreme Court erred when they decided to gut the AMA Principles of Medical Ethics two decades ago. Their desire to lower health care costs by promoting competition was perhaps well intentioned but overzealous. Their goal of applying free market economics to health care could have and should have included not excluded Hippocratic ethics.

The glaring void caused by the absence of the Hippocratic Oath from the AMA's Principles of Medical Ethics has been corrected with the adoption of new Section VIII, which states, "A physician shall, while caring for a patient, regard responsibility to the patient as paramount."

Why is this important? Section VIII can guide physicians in their daily interactions with patients, insurance companies and the government. It also should help restore patient trust in the medical profession. It might even offer guidance to the courts in their decisions on the ever-increasing number of cases that deal with managed care financial incentives and the conflicts of interest that they produce in physicians.

❧

Hippocratic Oath: "I swear by Apollo ... and Aesculapius that ... I ... will follow that system of regimen which, according to my ability and judgment, I consider for the benefit of my patients, and abstain from whatever is deleterious ..."

Section 6: 1975 **AMA Principles of Medical Ethics:** A physician should not dispose of his services under terms or conditions which tend to interfere with or impair the free and complete exercise of his medical judgment and skill or tend to cause a deterioration of the quality of medical care.

Part Two

Managed Care Escapes Regulation and Accountability

Wrap-Up—1993

Strategy For The Future

St. Louis Metropolitan Medicine
December 1993

- *Do away with ERISA*
- *Introduce legislation that will guarantee freedom of choice in the doctor-patient relationship*
- *Require accountability for employers and insurance companies*

What strategy should organized medicine take in the future with regard to health system reform?

To answer this question, we must first determine the cause of the current upheaval in health care delivery which has shaken the house of medicine to its very foundation. Specifically, we must determine why the corporate takeover of medicine began even before the Clinton administration health plan was on the table.

An obscure article in the *AM News* (Nov. 1, 1993) best explains why in 1993 corporate medicine finally decided to take charge of the medical profession. The article begins: "A change in accounting rules has accomplished something health care inflation didn't. As a result of huge write-offs taken this year for future retiree health benefits, for the first time, American companies are facing serious scrutiny of their care spending from board members and shareholders."

"This new accountability is driving employers to take

drastic steps to rein in health care spending: *eliminating indemnity coverage, restricting workers' choice of physicians, and forming provider networks.* Much of this frenzied activity can be traced to a new accounting rule, FASB 106, which requires companies to provide financial reserves to cover retiree health benefits for the first quarter of 1993. The resulting write-down in health care costs is a staggering $115 billion for the 50 largest firms in fiscal year 1992 alone ... FASB 106 will likely add $200-$300 billion for the rest of the Fortune 500 companies ... FASB 106 forces firms to justify their health care spending to shareholders for the first time. This new pressure is driving companies to demand competitive prices from doctors and hospitals."

So finally ... we have the explanation of why corporate America has chosen this time for its takeover of medicine. The immediate cause is—of all things—a simple new accounting rule, FASB 106. Corporate CEOs for the first time are now accountable to shareholders to hold medical costs in line. Previously they were able to confront their costs on a day-to-day, month-to-month basis.

We should, however, not feel undue sympathy for the plight of the corporate CEOs. As you will soon discover, this new accountability of CEOs to shareholders on health care costs is not matched by a corresponding accountability for their employees' health.

Another obscure article, this from the back pages of *The Wall Street Journal* (Oct. 25, 1993), is even more astonishing. It describes how corporate American can take just about whatever steps it chooses to cut costs and change the way in which health care is delivered in the marketplace without fearing scrutiny or interference from state and federal regulations. This article, titled "Employees Find There Is Little Recourse When Denied Care by Company

Health Plans," discusses Employees Retirement Income Security Act under which 60 percent of U.S. employees receive their health care. If you think that only lawyers, accountants, actuaries and government administrators would be interested in something as dull sounding as ERISA, think again! This law has permitted corporations at their own whim to turn medical care upside down. It drastically affects how you and I practice medicine.

People who buy individual health insurance plans are protected by state laws that prohibit insurers from unfairly denying claims, arbitrarily withholding treatment, or cutting off coverage if the policyholder becomes ill. If the insurer violates these state laws and regulations, policyholders can sue for benefits and damages. Under ERISA, employees are not protected. *ERISA is exempt from state laws. In addition, there are no federal laws pertaining to unfair insurance practices or insurance company malpractice.* A Labor Department spokesman said that the majority of the 180,000 complaints it received last year were about ERISA health plans.

The article cites cases where health plan administrators disagreed with the patients' doctors. In one instance, a plan administrator sent a patient who was eight months pregnant home without the treating physician's approval. When the fetus died, the patient sued the plan administrators. Because of ERISA, the lower court and appellate court threw out the suit.

Another example, which occurred in Redlands, Calif., was the case of premature twins born with serious illnesses. Hospital costs for the care of these infants soared to $450,000. The insurance company denied the claim because, according to them, the infants were "born with a preexisting condition." Under ERISA, the hospital and doctors could not recover their costs. (At last, we have learned how managed care achieves its vaunted savings! Don't pay the doctors and hospitals, by deciding, after the fact, that an expensive illness is not covered!) Many of you have had similar experiences, albeit not as dramatic, where insurance companies have denied claims arbitrarily, or engaged in the practice of medicine dictating patient care contrary to professional judgment.

Until I learned about ERISA, I naively believed, as do most citizens, that in America everyone is accountable.

Certainly, we doctors are accountable as no other profession. We are accountable under the law, not only to our patients, but also to a long list of federal, state and hospital regulations. We are also accountable to managed care plans, HMOs and PPOs sponsored by large corporations; the very plans which under ERISA are accountable to no one. But, in corporate America, employers and their insurance company handmaidens have unlimited and unchecked power.

What is going on here?

The founders of our country would be shocked if they knew about ERISA. The founders knew firsthand about the tyranny associated with unlimited power. They had suffered personally, religious, political and economic persecution, as a result of the unchecked power of European monarchs. That is why they constructed a government with checks and balances and separation of power. But Congress, almost 200 years later has forgotten the lessons of history. It has ignored the concepts of the founders.

In 1974, Congress created ERISA and exempted it from state law. The thinking of Congress was that unchecked by a myriad of often conflicting state laws, the companies could save money and afford to be more generous with employee benefits. Congress "trusted" the employers to do right by their employees. Perhaps the employers did "do right" for their employees in the past, but no more. The founders would have been very suspicious of the unchecked power granted to corporations in 1974, and they would have predicted what is happening two decades later. We should not be surprised at the actions of Congress in exempting ERISA from regulation. Congress has also exempted itself from every major law of the land for over two decades. That is why we, as citizens back home, are subject to so many oppressive laws.

No wonder corporate America can do what it pleases in order to cut costs. No wonder corporate America can force employees into health care plans such as HMOs against their will. No wonder corporate America can deny freedom of choice of physicians to their employees. No wonder corporate America can force physicians to join HMOs, when physicians are only willing to join PPOs. No wonder corporations can boldly deny claims and medical treatment to their employees. No wonder corporate America can literally get away with murder. No wonder corporate America paints a rosy picture of how they have cut medical costs more efficiently without sacrificing quality. Under ERISA, no one can challenge them. Under ERISA, corporations are immune to the normal constraints of law under which the rest of us operate. Can you imagine how corporate America and the health insurance industry would react even if a small portion of the 180,000 yearly complaints to the Labor Department about health care plans were translated into lawsuits? (Believe me, I am not generally a supporter of lawsuits as a way to settle differences or disputes.)

George Orwell was wrong! In his book, "1984," Big Brother was government. But ten years later in 1994, it is not government Big Brother that we have to fear, it is corporate Big Brother!

Employee advocates, consumer groups, insurance regulators, and states' attorneys general have all criticized ERISA. There are many other Americans who are becoming aware of the flaws in ERISA.

Congress tried to change the ERISA law last summer in order to allow states to initiate health system reform. No serious state health system reform can be enacted without an ERISA waiver. At the last minute, ERISA waivers were cancelled for Hawaii, Maryland, Minnesota and Oregon. An unholy alliance of big corporations, health insurers and, unexpectedly, organized labor fought hard against congressional waivers. The Clinton administration has been ambivalent on this issue. President Bill Clinton is reported to have not wanted to get into an ERISA fight.

What does this mean to organized medicine? As a strategy to achieve its goals and have meaningful input into health system reform, whether on a state or national level, the SLMMS, MSMA and AMA have to join the battle for ERISA waivers, repeal, or modification. If the SLMMS wishes to achieve passage of its eight legislative goals, ERISA will have to go.

Right now corporate America is a monopsony a monopoly of purchasers. Under ERISA, corporate America can thumb its nose at all the values which we as Americans cherish, such as freedom of choice. The state legislators are sympathetic to the goals of the medical profession and would rein in corporate America if they were legally empowered to do so. Perhaps, as recommended by Nobel Laureate conservative economist, Milton Friedman, corporations should just get out of the health insurance business altogether.

The debate on ERISA has just begun. Discussion is under way. It will be just a matter of time until ERISA is modified, repealed or waived. It is just a matter of time until corporate power is checked, and medical insurance companies are held accountable for denying claims and practicing medicine.

The Time Has Arrived To Repeal The McCarran-Ferguson Act

The Insurance Industry—The last bastion of privilege in our society
St. Louis Metropolitan Medicine
November 1994

Why, one might ask, write articles about laws such as ERISA and now an article on the McCarran-Ferguson Act? The answer is that laws, or more accurately the absence of laws, have permitted the big business/insurance industry coalition to take over medicine.

The reader may recall that earlier this year when the democratically elected governor of the state of Missouri introduced a health reform bill, a lobbyist for General American Life Insurance Company challenged the bill on legal grounds. He maintained that the reform bill, through its community rating provision requiring all companies — regardless of size — to pay equally for health care, violated the ERISA preemption. He threatened to sue in the Eighth Federal Circuit Court and boasted that General American would prevail in such a suit. The governor and his supporters backed down because General American probably *would* have prevailed in court. Regardless of what one thinks about the governor's health reform bill, the principle was established that the insurance industry and their big business bosses can thwart the will of the governor, the state legislature and the citizens of the state of Missouri, because of a poorly written federal law ERISA (Employer Retirement Income Security Act of 1974), which exempts the insurance industry from state regulations.

Another law that enhances the power of the insurance industry and supposedly immunizes it against federal antitrust regulations is the McCarran-Ferguson Act of 1945. Federal antitrust laws prohibit price fixing and monopolistic practices.

Did Congress really intend to exempt the insurance industry from antitrust regulations? The answer is emphatically no. The Congress did not intend to exempt the insurance industry from antitrust, but to grant states the right to regulate and tax insurance companies.

The AMA policy compendium of 1994 (Edition 180, 975, p. 184), titled "Insurance Industry Anti-trust Exemption" delves into the history of the McCarran-Ferguson Act. The AMA Board of Trustees' Report DD (191) comes to a very important and surprising conclusion.

The McCarran-Ferguson Act specifically states *"... that the Sherman Act, the Clayton Act and the Federal Trade Commission Act (all of the federal antitrust laws) 'shall be applicable to the business of insurance, to the extent that such business is not regulated by state law.'"* McCarran-Ferguson then, specifically excludes acts of boycott coercion or intimidation from the state. These will remain subject to federal antitrust laws.

In plain English, this means Congress intended the states to write antitrust regulations and if they did not do so, federal laws would apply. As one might expect, the states, for the most part, either never wrote or enforced antitrust laws. For acts of coercion, intimidation or boycott, federal antitrust law would continue to take precedence over state laws. But McCarran-Ferguson erected a psychological barrier that stands until the present day, preventing effective challenge to insurance company antitrust immunity.

From 1945 to 1979, the McCarran-Ferguson Act withstood all legal challenges. The case, which tore down the walls on insurance company antitrust exemption under McCarran, has major implications for the medical profession. In the case of *Group Life and Health Insurance vs. Royal Drug,* commonly known as "Royal Drug," a group of independent pharmacists sued Group Life and Health Insurance (a Blue Shield plan) and defendant pharmacies for antitrust violations. Group Life entered into exclusive financial arrangements with three Texas pharmacies, which from a practical standpoint, eliminated or severely reduced the business of nonparticipating pharmacies. The nonparticipating pharmacies claimed that the agreement caused policyholders to "boycott" them and that the insurance company engaged in price fixing and exclusionary practices. These suggestions, if true, amounted to violations of the Sherman Act.

The Supreme Court agreed that the allegations, if true, *did* violate the Sherman Act and remanded the case back to the federal court. The principle had been established by the U.S. Supreme Court that the defendant insurance companies could not, as they had tried to do, claim antitrust exemption under McCarran-Ferguson.

The Royal Drug case anticipated, by over a decade, exactly what is happening today to physicians all over the United States. It anticipated what has already happened in Minneapolis/St. Paul and what is about to happen right here in St. Louis. Insurance companies and large corporations make financial arrangements with a certain group of participating doctors. Nonparticipating doctors are excluded. The exclusion of doctors from these plans could be interpreted as an illegal boycott. The insurance companies' transactions with the participating physicians could be interpreted as price fixing. This is similar to what was alleged in the Royal Drug case, and this level of behavior was what the Supreme Court specifically states was *not* exempted by the McCarran-Ferguson Act.

To my knowledge, no physician group has ever challenged the insurance industry on this issue, probably because of the mistaken and universally held notion that under McCarran-Ferguson, insurance companies are exempt from antitrust regulation.

The supposed insurance company exemption from antitrust activities is derided and ridiculed by almost every segment of our society, not just physicians. The president of the United States, our elected representatives in state and federal government, members of the administration (including the Justice Department), federal and state insurance regulators and the National Association of Attorneys General, all support the overthrow of McCarran. They are supported by consumer organizations. One consumer spokesperson said that, "Repeal of McCarran would be a positive step for consumers because antitrust exemptions mean higher prices and poorer service. McCarran is an act that has long outlived its uselessness." (Pun intended.)

A bill before Congress now, HR 9, the Insurance Competition Pricing Act of 1993, would specifically ban insurance companies from price fixing, allocating and monopolizing markets. This would be in addition to the already banned practices of coercion, intimidation and boycott.

The Clinton Health Plan, Title 5, Subtitled F, as well as other health care proposals, provides that the McCarran-Ferguson Act no longer apply to the delivery of health insurance.

Currently, American Medical Association policy does not call for repeal of McCarran-Ferguson, even though resolutions calling for its repeal have been introduced in the House of Delegates in the past.

In this period of health system reform, the time is right for McCarran repeal. Large insurance companies and their big business allies have never been more brazen in carving up markets, fixing prices, boycotting doctors, and intimidating and coercing patients, as well as physicians. The medical profession has allies among the public, on both sides of the aisle in Congress, and in the Administration, who are united to bring down McCarran.

In my opinion, most of the evils that we physicians have encountered in the corporate/insurance industry takeover of medicine would never have been permitted to occur, if the insurance industry and their allies operated under the rule of law. Their lawless behavior, their abuse of power under McCarran-Ferguson and ERISA, has not only resulted in monopolizing the markets, price fixing, unfair insurance practices and poor quality patient care for which they are not accountable, but has allowed them to thwart the will of the people in enacting health system reform and universal coverage for all Americans.

To top it off, while the insurance industry considers itself exempt from antitrust, it has the audacity (supported by big business and now the American Hospital Association) to oppose antitrust relief for the oppressed medical profession.

The time has come, long overdue, for the insurance industry to operate under the yoke of the law, just like everyone else in our society.

The Medical Marketplace Needs More, Not Less, Regulation:

Managed Care Strives to Escape Accountability

Missouri Medicine
March 1995

Today the buzzwords for controlling medical costs are "let the marketplace work," or "the marketplace is already working, we don't need government interference." Most of the time these words are spoken by representatives of the for-profit managed care HMOs and their big business backers.

Physicians as small businessmen are often sympathetic to this point of view. Furthermore, as members of perhaps the most over-regulated profession in the nation, many physicians have joined the chorus in supporting an unfettered marketplace. But does our medical profession really understand what is happening in the marketplace? While physicians are over-regulated, the insurance industry and particularly the for-profit HMOs are hardly regulated at all. In our so-called free market, physicians are at a marked disadvantage in dealing with insurance companies.

The following is a list of major areas where the insurance industry and their patrons — the large corporations — have been able to escape accountability.

Anti-trust: The McCarran-Ferguson Act exempts the insurance industry from Federal anti-trust laws which apply to almost all other major U.S. businesses. Anti-trust regulation is left to the states. The states often apply these regulations unevenly and often lack the financial resources and legal expertise to pursue anti-trust violations vigorously.

Physicians, on the other hand, feel the heavy hand of government anti-trust regulations. If two physicians even dare to discuss the price of an office visit, they can be hauled into court and fined. Meanwhile, large HMO oligopolies carve up markets and virtually dictate reimbursement to the medical profession.

ERISA (Employee Retirement Income Security Act): ERISA is the federal law which applies to companies, labor unions, and trade associations that self-insure. From 60-65 percent of all employees in the United States are covered under ERISA. Many physicians are familiar with the fact that in order to initiate health care reform, states need ERISA waivers. But few members of our profession are aware that employers and their third party administrators—the for-profit HMOs—are not accountable and not liable under ERISA for acts of medical negligence or for unfair insurance practices. Two famous court cases—McGann and Corcoran—confirmed ERISA's fight to pre-empt state insurance regulations.

The most flagrant and widely known case of unfair insurance practices is the McGann case. In 1988, John McGann of Houston contracted AIDS. *After* he ran up bills totaling $5,000, his employer changed the plan and limited medical expenses for AIDS to $5,000. McGann sued his employer for discriminatory practices. The Federal Circuit and Appellate courts both ruled that under

ERISA, his employer had a perfect right to change the plan at any time. The U.S. Supreme Court refused to hear the case.

The Corcoran case from Alabama illustrates that patients injured by insurance companies' utilization practices cannot obtain justice. In 1992, Florence Corcoran was eight months pregnant. Her obstetrician recommended that she remain in the hospital because of medical problems associated with her pregnancy. To save money, the insurance company utilization review managers refused to pay for further hospitalization. She was discharged against her doctor's advice; the fetus went into distress and died. Corcoran sued the insurance company in Federal court. The court ruled that although the outcome was not just, under ERISA Corcoran did not have a valid claim.

These court decisions granted self-insured corporations and their HMO third party administrators the right to treat the health of their employees as they see fit, with full immunity from liability.

Hold harmless clauses: As if ERISA were not enough to ensure their immunity from liability, the managed care insurance companies have their physician providers sign hold harmless clauses. The managed care HMOs want to "manage" patient care but if something goes wrong, guess who is left holding the bag. It is certainly not the insurance company who is actually engaged in the micromanaging of patient care, but it is the doctor who signed the hold harmless clause.

If the government micromanaged care like the for-profit HMOs, every doctor in the country would be screaming to his or her legislator about the intrusiveness of Big Brother. When the private insurance coalition dictates how physicians should treat their patients in a "free market," for some unknown reason there is hardly a murmur of protest.

Medical standards, guidelines, outcome studies, physician profiling and de-selection: Insurance companies are developing their own practice parameters, utilization review, outcome studies and physician profiling. The software for these activities is already in place. The for-profit HMOs do not use guidelines concerned with quality of care, which are developed by specialty societies or government licensing agencies. They develop their own guidelines because their primary goals are cutting costs and increasing profits.

Consider the hurdles, which the student must overcome to become a practicing physician. There is pre-med, acceptance to and graduation from a licensed medical school, state licensure, residency program, and board certification. In this entire process, which can take from 12 to 16 years of an aspiring doctor's life, professional organizations such as medical schools, government licensing agents, academic medical centers and specialty societies, determine who can become a physician and how and what he or she may practice. Now, all over America, for-profit HMOs have usurped the traditional role of academic medical centers, professional organizations and government licensing agencies, to dictate how physicians must practice and care for patients. If a physician does not follow the guidelines established by the insurance companies, which are often based on economic necessities (economic credentialing), he or she may be de-selected from the plan and have no patients to treat. If the physician complains that he or she was acting in the best medical interest of the patient, there is no independent appeals process. The physician can be kicked out of the plan for complaining.

Failure to inform enrollees of the details of operation of the managed care plan: Presently managed care plan are not required to inform enrollees about details of the plans' operation. Enrollees are kept in the dark about physician financial incentives to under-serve patients, e.g., the gatekeeper withhold. Enrollees are not informed in plain English about the plan's exclusions, limitations of physician choice, co-payments, co-insurance, referral and treatment options. In other words, in the world of managed care, there are no truth in lending, truth in packaging, or truth in labeling laws as there are in almost every other major U.S. industry.

The so-called free market can best be described as a competitive sport, like football, basketball or baseball. When the ball is thrown in play, the side which is most competitive gains the victory. "May the best man win" is the motto accepted by most Americans. But in all sporting events, the contestants compete according to strict rules, so that one side does not have an advantage over the other. This is why we so often hear today the cliché, "level the playing field". The problem in the medical marketplace is that the insurance companies and their big business backers have come to the contest with their own set of rules. And they often change the rules in the middle of the game.

The domination of the market by the payers raises the age-old question of what is the proper function of government. The answer is that the proper role of government is to set and enforce the rules of the game to ensure that the contest is fair, so that the final outcome in the marketplace is the best quality product at the lowest cost.

In framing our republic, the founding fathers did not discuss "free markets." They knew from their study of history that the most important function of government is to prevent tyranny by limiting power. That is why our Constitution established checks and balances and separation of powers. Checks and balances and limitation of power apply not just to the structure of government, but to the private sector and to the marketplace, including the medical marketplace.

According to historian Joseph Ellis in his book, "Passionate Sage," John Adams (signer of the Declaration of Independence, second president of the Unites States, and a leading intellectual light of the Federalists) never believed in the benign operation of the marketplace. As an old Puritan, he understood human nature. Without regulation, the marketplace will degenerate into a jungle where the strong will dominate the weak. Tyranny will ensure and society will break down. James Madison, father of the U.S. Constitution, agreed with Adams that government is the guarantor, not the threat, to liberty. That is why the government regulates the stock market, banks, savings & loans associations, the automobile industry, and just about every other American industry.

But the insurance industry and their corporate customers want to remain exempt from regulations. At the recent Missouri House of Representatives' hearings, the business-insurance lobby testified against the Patient Fairness Act sponsored by the MSMA. Among those who testified against the Act were Blue Cross/Blue Shield, CIGNA, Missouri Chamber of Commerce, National Federation of Independent Business and General American. It is not difficult to understand why they would be against regulations which would make their industry as accountable as every other industry in the United States and as accountable as the medical profession.

The managed care industry has put forth a host of arguments in opposition to the Patient Fairness Act. For example, they call the Act a doctor-protection act because it contains an any willing provider clause. (It does not contain such a clause.) But basically all of their arguments can be boiled down to three words: *avoidance of accountability*. The insurance industry knows that if it were held accountable, it would no longer achieve its so-called cost savings; it would no longer be able to dominate the market and reap enormous profits.

All citizens, including our elected legislators, the medical profession and even businessmen and insurance executives should understand that regulation—not the over-regulation which our nation has recently experienced—is a necessity for our democratic society to function properly. According to the framers, accountability and limitation of power comes first and is more important than the unregulated, so-called free market. No one stands above the law. That's the American way of doing things.

Can American Democracy and The Profession of Medicine Survive The Giant Managed Care Oligopolies?

Justice Louis D. Brandeis and "The Curse of Bigness"
Missouri Medicine
June 1995

As health system reform proceeds in the marketplace, the insurance companies grow larger and larger, securing even greater economic and political power.

The founders of our nation knew well the lessons of history—the uncontrolled concentration of power always leads to abuse. They fashioned a Constitution with checks and balances and separation of powers, which prevent government from usurping the liberties of a free people. But the founders never addressed the problem of the concentration of power in the hands of large corporations because mega-corporations simply did not exist at that time. The American economy at the time that the Constitution was written was mainly agrarian.

After the Civil War, in the late 19th and early 20th centuries with the Industrial Revolution in full swing, corporations or trusts as they were called at that time grew to enormous size. They were controlled by a small number of financiers who often served on interlocking directorates.

There were many leaders in government and society

at large who viewed oligopolies (the concentration of economic and political power in the hands of a few) as a threat to American democracy. The most outspoken and influential opponent of trusts and the threat they posed to a democratic society was Justice Louis D. Brandeis (1856-1941). He wrote a famous essay on the trusts titled "The Curse of Bigness." He fought the trusts in the courts and was involved in the creation of the Federal Trade Commission and the Clayton Anti-Trust Act.

Brandeis criticized the trusts for four major reasons. One, they held too much concentrated power; two, they were inefficient; three, they were responsible for the deterioration of quality; and four, they did not permit the development of free, autonomous individuals who were so necessary for the maintenance of democracy.

Let us examine each of these items with reference to the managed care mega insurance companies.

1) The concentration of corporate power in Brandeis' time was enormous. Today in the health care sector of our economy, we see s similar pattern of concentration of wealth and power. Best Insurance Report (Life-Health 1993) showed the following net worth of the five largest insurance companies:

Prudential	**154.1 billion**
Met Life	**118.1 billion**
Aetna	**67.1 billion**
Cigna	**47.1 billion**
Travelers	**34.2 billion**

The assets of these insurance companies equal or exceed the GDP of many nations.

These insurance companies not only wield economic power, they wield political power. One has to look no further than to the recent events that took place in the Missouri

State legislature. When the Missouri State Medical Association introduced a bill regulating the quality of care delivered by the insurance industry (The Patient Fairness Act), the insurance industry and their big business patrons sent an "army" of lobbyists to Jefferson City, Mo. This bill passed handily in the Senate. It had a reasonable chance of passing the House, but it never came out of committee in the House because the insurance industry controlled the committee to which it was referred. These well-heeled lobbyists contribute not only to the election campaigns of legislators, but they have the resources to offer jobs to legislators and their families. Is it any wonder that the average American is cynical about government? Some political scientists and pundits describe our government as a "cashocracy," not a democracy, because the power of the special interest has destroyed the one man, one vote concept, which is so essential to the maintenance of our democracy.

2) The inefficiency of large corporations. Brandeis held that huge size of corporations produced inefficiency. Because of his corporate law practice, he had firsthand knowledge of the financing of the trusts. He knew about the dark side of corporate finance. He knew how corporate managers manipulated figures to show increased shareholder profits. He knew about the waste, inefficiency and corruption that can occur in trusts.

Economists have roundly criticized Brandeis for his economic views on bigness. They think that as an economist Brandeis was naive despite his mastery of the most intricate accounting data in corporate finance.

Economists believe that bigness by virtue of vertical integration and economy of scale (sound familiar?) is efficient because it produces low prices for the consumer. Economists hold that Brandeis failed to distinguish between *central industries* like automobiles, steel and chemicals, and *peripheral industries* like furniture, lumber and apparel manufacturing. The former by their nature always develop into huge vertically integrated industries, whereas the latter have never evolved in that manner.

The medical industry has traditionally been a cottage industry-with a few notable exceptions like Kaiser Permanente. In the present evolving medical marketplace, economists, business school professors, and public policy makers are forcing vertical integration and economy of scale on the health care industry through managed care HMOs. Their rationale is that the medical care industry is a *central industry* not a *peripheral industry*. But the basic assumption that large HMOs whether vertically integrated or not, are economical may be fallacious. Consider the following:

1. The 1984 Puget Sound/Rand Study, the last double blind randomized, controlled study comparing the cost of fee-for-service and HMOs, showed the HMOs were not less expensive than fee-for-service plans with modest cost sharing.

2. The 1993 exhaustive General Accounting Office review of all studies comparing HMOs and traditional insurance concluded that there was no scientific evidence that HMOs were less expensive than traditional insurance plans.

3. In 1994, two independent studies, one by the Mathematica Corporation and one by the GAO showed that HMOs were actually more expensive than traditional insurance in the Medicare population.

4. Joseph Newhouse, a Harvard economist, reported

in *Health Affairs* (Winter, 1994) that the per capita growth rate of health care in this country has remained relatively steady through 1993. The average growth rate per capita is 3-4 percent. This is in contrast to the reports that premiums charged to business have not increased significantly over the past few years due to the introduction of managed care. For a variety of reasons, Newhouse says that the data provided by big business is not an adequate indicator of the facts. Employers have cut benefits; employees are a healthier population; and furthermore 40 percent of health care financing is public.

The high administrative costs of HMOs also contribute to waste. In California, *A.M. News* (5/1/95) reports that administrative costs of private HMOs for Medicaid patients were much greater than the administrative costs for the state. HMO costs were 16 percent on an average, and state administrative costs were 2 percent. Salaries for HMO administrators have soared out of sight. On a national level, cash and stock dividends to the CEOs of the seven biggest for-profit HMOs averaged $7 million last year.

Administrative costs for HMOs across the United States range from 27.1 percent (U.S. Health Care) to 16.5 percent (Pacific Care Health Systems). These facts, contrary to the views of the economists, business school professors, and public policy experts, attest to Brandeis' theories that bigness does not always produce efficiency.

3) Brandeis believed that the third major problem of bigness was that it usually resulted in deterioration of quality. According to one political scientist, trusts at the turn of the century were perceived something akin to "acts of God." Their existence was thought by many to be "inevitable and good."

Today, HMO operators hype consolidation and integrations as a means of lowering price and improving quality, just as the steel and railroad magnates of Brandeis' time claimed for their industries. Were he alive, Brandeis probably would not buy the arguments of today's HMO operators any more than he bought the arguments of big business 80 years ago. With an uncanny talent for analyzing corporate financial statements, and by refusing to accept uncritically the data presented by big business, Brandeis demonstrated how trusts ossified, suppressed competition, stifled innovation and ended up producing poor quality products at higher prices. A recent example of this phenomenon is the U.S. auto industry prior to the introduction of foreign competition.

The HMOs pride themselves on the quality of care they deliver. They have their own quality assurance organization called the National Committee on Quality Assurance. The NCQA is not a truly independent organization; it is run by the trade association that it is supposed to regulate. The AMA selects one member who serves on the NCQA board.

Other quality indicators for HMOs are that they check the charts for content and legibility. They encourage preventative health programs in order to prevent serious costly illnesses from developing, and in order to further enhance their image of quality, HMOs send out surveys which usually conclude that 90-95 percent of their enrollees are happy with their HMOs and happy with their physicians. I have no quarrel with these activities. They are activities that physicians have always engaged in and are nothing new. But basically they are screening types of activities.

But what happens if a patient develops a costly and

serious illness, the kind of illness that many of us were trained to treat? That's when the managed care HMOs can become downright nasty.

About 65 percent of all employees in the United States are covered under the federal Employee Retirement Income Security Act. State insurance commissions have no jurisdiction over these plans and, because the ERISA law was poorly written, neither does the federal government. So it turns out that ERISA plans, which are basically synonymous with the large for-profit HMOs, are not accountable for poor medical practices to anyone. History shows what that always leads to.

It is no surprise then that the National Association of Insurance Commissioners issued a white paper in March 1995, which called for ERISA reform. In their conclusion, they stated the following: "The diverse facts of ERISA's failure to protect the interests of health care consumers are widely reported frequently as isolated incidents. The large number of reported cases, thousands of complaints, and hundreds of media stories, document the hurt and despair of many individuals."

The same white paper contained the words of the judge who heard the Corcoran case where a woman with complications of pregnancy was sent home, against the advice of her obstetrician, by the utilization review board of a large HMO. While the mother was at home, the fetus developed distress and died. Corcoran sued the insurance company, but could not obtain redress of her grievance under ERISA law. The judge, in acknowledging the injustice of his own opinion, had the following to say about ERISA (and about the utilization review committees of the for-profit HMOs which are covered under the ERISA law):

[ERISA] removes an important check on the thousands of medical decisions routinely made in the burgeoning utilization review system ... there is no deterrence for substandard medical decision-making ... bad medical judgments will end up being cost-free ... ERISA plans will have one less incentive to seek out the company that can deliver both high quality services and reasonable prices.

These are strong words. The dire predictions of the judge have come to pass in California. The California Medical Association and consumer organizations have introduced a record 80 bills trying to regulate managed care companies. A spokesperson for the CMA said (*A.M. News*, May 8, 1995), "We see a cumulative effect of thousands of patients who have been suffering and fighting the system without any rights. Consumer outcry has really come to a head." Two high-profile judgments may have contributed to this public outcry. One was an $89.3 million jury award last year to the family of a patient who was refused by an HMO, the cost of covering an autologous bone marrow transplant to treat her breast cancer. The other was a $500,000 fine levied by the state in 1994 against another California HMO for refusing to provide a pediatric surgical specialist for a young girl diagnosed with Wilms' tumor.

When we talk about quality of care, whom are we to believe—on the one hand the large managed care companies or on the other hand the National Association of Insurance Commissioners, the courts, the California Medical Association and consumer groups? In one scenario, one of the parties must not be telling the truth. The reader may decide for himself or herself who that party is.

In another scenario, it is possible that all parties to this dispute are correct. How is this possible? It is estimated that in the United States, 5-10 percent of the population consumes 50 percent of medical resources. When managed care insurance companies' surveys show that 90-95 percent of their members are happy with their plan, the conclusion may be true. The 90-95 percent who are happy with their HMO may be the ones who do not have a serious illness. The 5-10 percent who are unhappy may, for the most part, be patients who have serious and costly illnesses. The state insurance commissioners, the courts, the CMA, and the consumer organizations are mainly up in arms over patients with serious illnesses who were denied treatment or mistreated by the HMOs.

If managed care were required to care for all the genuinely sick patients we see in our practices and if they were made accountable to the American public through the courts by repeal of ERISA, in my opinion much of their so-called cost savings would evaporate.

4) Brandeis' fourth major objection to big business was that it deprived citizens of liberty or "manhood" as he called it. By manhood, Brandeis meant a free autonomous human being. Brandeis believed that democracy is fragile and cannot survive if its citizens are not free.

Brandeis' statements on freedom may sound a bit corny to some readers, but let's look at what's happened to freedom for employees and physicians under managed care.

Employers herd their employees like cattle into HMOs. Employees often lose the freedom to choose their own doctors with whom they have built a relationship over many years. They may be forced to change physicians every year or two because their employer chooses a different plan for economic reasons. They often cannot see the specialists of their choice. They certainly cannot see any specialist without first getting approval of a primary care "gatekeeper." Even the specialists on the list approved by the employer's HMO may not be available to the employee because the gatekeeper's withhold may be affected unless he sends patients to a certain group of specialists who are credentialed as "economically more efficient." When the patient goes to a primary care physician and needs an EKG, chest x-ray or laboratory blood test, he or she must traipse all over the city—sometimes in bad weather—to obtain tests that they could have more conveniently obtained in their physician's office. A small, but significant, number of patients (10-20 percent—no one really knows how many) simply never obtain these because of the hassles involved. The HMO manager mandates these rules in the name of "efficiency."

If the patients are denied freedom of choice and must do what they are told, physicians are not much better off. In order to be accepted by the HMO, physicians must sign a "hold harmless" agreement. They must relieve the managed care organization of liability, even though the managed care organization may directly micromanage and interfere with physician decision-making. HMOs often require physicians to sign "gag orders," prohibiting them from saying negative things about the operating practices of the plan, and physicians must promise not to recommend other physicians in rival organizations. If, because of their conscience, physicians speak negatively about the practices of the plan, they can be kicked out or as it is euphemistically termed, deselected. One can only wonder who the doctor is working for—the patient or the insurance company.

Doctors today are working in a climate of fear. An atmosphere of corporate "big brotherism" prevails.

Brandeis was right—people working in such an environment will not develop the necessary liberties that a democracy requires. They will simply do what they are told. Witness the "efficient" totalitarian regimes in Germany, Japan, Italy and Russia in the 1930s and 1940s.

When one considers all of the potentially harmful effects of corporate bigness, is it really worthwhile for the United States to embark on the managed care experiment which is being forced down the throats of the American public and the medical profession? Even if there are some small cost savings, is it worth the effort?

No one has given a more eloquent answer to this question than Louis D. Brandeis. In his testimony before the Senate committee on Interstate Commerce in 1911, Brandeis spoke the following words:

"The ill effects of bigness weigh heavily on both men and things. By their by-products shall ye know the trusts. Study them, through the spectacles of people's rights and people's interests ... when you do that you will realize the extraordinary perils to our institutions which attend the trust. ... Aside from whether a corporation has exceeded the power of 'greatest economic efficiency' or not, it may be too large to be tolerated among the people who desire to be free."

⌘

Justice Louis D. Brandeis

Justice Louis D. Brandeis is sometimes referred to as the Thomas Jefferson of industrial democracy. The young Brandeis bore a close physical resemblance to Lincoln, according to persons who knew both men. His colleagues on the Supreme Court and President Woodrow Wilson referred to him in conversation as

"Isaiah" after the Old Testament prophet. Brandeis' beliefs and actions were in keeping with the principles of individual freedom and equality held by all three of these individuals.

Brandeis was well qualified to understand the inner workings of corporations. He had firsthand knowledge as an eminently successful corporation lawyer. His uniqueness lay in the fact that, despite representing the rich and powerful, he had a strong social conscience. After becoming wealthy from his law practice, he came to champion the cause of the workingman. He won a landmark case obtaining shorter working hours for employees. He successfully battled the president of the United States, William Howard Taft, and one of his Cabinet members on an issue of granting mineral rights in Alaska. Because of his advocacy of the public interest and the rights of the common citizen, he became known as the people's lawyer. He never accepted a fee for his work in this area of the law.

His greatest accomplishments, however, were in his opposition to, and the regulation of, the giant monopolies or trusts that existed in the early decades of this century. Although he was quite popular with the public, he developed many powerful enemies in corporate America. When he was nominated for the United States Supreme Court by President Woodrow Wilson, no less than seven former presidents of the American Bar Association, including a previous president of the United States, William Howard Taft, wrote letters opposing the nomination, describing him as morally unfit for the job. His nomination to the

Supreme Court was confirmed despite this formidable opposition.

Brandeis' comments on the threats to democracy of the trust are germane to the mega for-profit HMOs which have mushroomed across the face of our nation in the past few years.

Managed Care Faces Ethical Showdown on Gag Rules

St. Louis Metropolitan Medicine
February 1997

Gag rules are one of the cornerstones of managed care's supposed cost savings. There are two kinds of gag rules. The first bans doctors from telling patients about all of their therapeutic options for treatment of serious and expensive illnesses. The second bans doctors from telling patients about physician financial incentives under managed care. These incentives include capitation, withholds, bonuses, and essentially place the physician at financial risk for patient care. Under these financial incentives the physician makes more money if he or she orders fewer tests and procedures, and makes fewer referrals to specialists.

The Health Care Finance Administration is to be commended for its recent ban on gag rules which forbid a doctor from telling Medicaid and Medicare patients all of their therapeutic options. The ban does not affect gag rules which prevent patients from learning about the financial incentives under which physicians work in managed care.

In Missouri, the recent report by The Joint Interim Committee on Managed Care also bans gag rules which forbid a doctor from telling a patient about all of the available therapeutic options. But, like the HCFA regulations, the ban does not cover gag rules pertaining to the financial incentives under which physicians work in managed care. The report states "These ... (capitation) ... arrangements should be deemed proprietary information and should not be publicly disclosed."

We have then a contradictory (if not ludicrous) situation where physician financial incentives are discussed openly and freely by government officials and the media, but are not to be disclosed directly to the public in their insurance contracts.

Why have managed care companies so fiercely resisted disclosure of the financial details of capitation? The answer is that managed care companies believe that this new and revolutionary method of paying physicians constitutes the foundation of their plan to cut medical costs (and incidentally enhance their own profits). Managed care fears that if the public learns about capitation and its attendant financial incentives to withhold care the entire managed care revolution could unravel.

Our country faces an ethical dilemma—whether to tell the public the truth and perhaps increase medical costs or whether to deceive the public and possibly cut medical costs.

The history of our nation dictates which course to follow.

The most calamitous event in our nation's history was the Civil War. If the average citizen is asked what the war was fought over the reply is usually slavery.

If an economist is asked the same question, he might well give a different answer. Many economists hold a unidimensional view of man as *homo economicus*. Human behavior is explained primarily in economic terms. The economists contend that at the time of the Civil War, slavery was no longer an efficient means of production. The institution of slavery was in the process of breaking down. According to this school of thought, the Civil War was fought over economic issues, not slavery.

In 1993, Donald Fogel, an economist from the University of Chicago, won the Nobel Prize in economics by proving that at the time of the Civil War, slavery was efficient. It was not disintegrating. The institution of slavery was producing lower consumer prices for cotton and other products. He published a four-volume study which concluded that slavery ended not because it was inefficient, but because it was "morally repugnant."

What has all this to do with gag rules?

Like slavery, gag rules are morally repugnant because their aim is to deceive the American public. Even if they produced lower consumer prices for medical services, they have no place in a free and open society. But the managed care industry has sold cost-conscious politicians on the importance of keeping financial incentives secret. The Clinton administration has stated that the financial incentives must remain proprietary if Medicare and Medicaid HMOs are to achieve their projected savings.

Recently, because of consumer concern over the potential harm which physician financial incentives might pose to patient care, HCFA, in part, reversed itself. As of Dec. 26, 1996, HCFA will require Medicare HMOs to provide beneficiaries a summary of their financial incentive arrangements with doctors if they request it. The new HCFA rules do not, in my opinion, go far enough because most beneficiaries are not sufficiently well informed to request the summary.

However, the public is eventually going to find out about physician financial incentives, regardless of gag clauses. And the managed care industry knows this.

The *Wall Street Journal*, Nov. 17, 1996, published an article reporting that the American Association of Health Plans, the trade association that represents about 1000 HMOs and managed care plans, has announced "a new initiative to curb the use of gag clauses." Under the initiative HMOs "will be expected to provide" some information on how their physicians are paid and how decisions are made about denying or approving medical care.

This change of heart on the part of managed care companies did not come about spontaneously. It came about because of widespread public criticism. The marketplace, including consumers, the media, public officials and concerned doctors (especially the AMA) spoke out loudly and clearly that they did not approve the gag rules.

In my opinion, this change of heart on gag rules is a move by the HMO industry to forestall any further Federal and state legislation on gag rules. Our elected officials should not allow managed care companies to police themselves on the important issue of gag clauses. They should pass strict laws outlawing these practices.

Politicians must understand that the managed care insurance companies, which introduced gag clauses in the first place, have little respect for the democratic principles of a free people. They must understand that these principles, many of which were forged on the bloody battlefields of the Civil and other wars, demand that when morality clashes with economics, morality must triumph.

Managed Care Bill Passes

Voice of the People Defeats HMO and Business Lobbies
St. Louis Metropolitan Medicine
July 1997

Managed care has been riding high. Despite media and public criticism of many of its practices, it has been essentially an unregulated industry. It has had free rein in issuing gag rules to doctors, and in denying or delaying tests, procedures, referrals and hospital admissions. Managed care also has operated without proper appeals mechanisms for both patients and physicians.

By enacting House Bill 335, which regulates managed care, the Missouri Legislature issued a strong rebuke to the HMO industry and its business backers. The bill engendered strong passions in those opposing and supporting it. When the House passed the final bill, members broke into spontaneous applause.

The invincibility of managed care in resisting regulation is being shattered all over the country as more and more states are enacting managed care laws. And nationally, new managed care regulations are being introduced.

Most readers are familiar with HB 335. Its salient points are listed in the accompanying box. The bill does not solve the managed care problem for most employed Missourians because it does not cover companies which self-insure their employees. These companies are covered under a national statute known as ERISA, which preempts all state regulations. ERISA covers about 50 to 60 percent of employed workers nationwide and in Missouri. But passage of HB 335 is certainly a first step in the right direction.

A politically powerful and wealthy lobby mobilized all its forces to defeat this bill. In St. Louis, this lobby represented the major insurance companies including the Blues and United Health Care; it also represented major business associations including the St. Louis Business Health Coalition, Civic Progress, and the Regional Commerce and Growth Association. It is important to understand the strategy and tactics of the HMO lobby because these interest groups may try to repeal HB 335 in the future. They certainly will oppose similar laws, which will be introduced nationally, which will apply to employees covered under ERISA.

The best description of HMO legislative strategies and tactics is by George Anders, a *Wall Street Journal* reporter. He recently wrote a book called "Health Against Wealth — HMOs and the Breakdown of Medical Trust."

In a chapter titled "The Best Lobbyists in America," Anders exposes managed care's plan of action. In 1995, at the time that the first national and state bills regulating HMOs were introduced, the national Blue Cross and Blue Shield Association went to pollster Gary Ferguson of American Viewpoint. Ferguson and associates found that, after talking with a number of focus groups composed of consumers and employees, the public preferred fee-for-service not HMOs as the best method for satisfying health care needs.

Ferguson warned that a fact-based campaign against proposed laws regulating managed care would lose. He went on to recommend, "visceral direct attacks against this legislation and its sponsors — and government involvement in general." In other words, Ferguson's message to the HMO lobbyists was: Avoid the truth and appeal to emotions. If this message sounds familiar, it is because, throughout history, these tactics have been used by demagogues, despots and dictators.

Ferguson, in his memo, then exhorts his clients to "Go after the AMA (American Medical Association) through surrogates." He identifies as example surrogates the Chamber of Commerce and the National Federation of Independent Business. These are the organizations which should hammer home the message of "government involvement ... higher costs ... bad for business ... rich doctors vs. consumers and employees ... matters that should be decided in the marketplace, not the legislature."

About two and one-half years ago, lobbyists for business associations successfully testified against the national AMA-sponsored Patient Protection Act using the exact techniques recommended by Ferguson. Shortly thereafter, at a Missouri legislative hearing, I heard for myself how business lobbyists testified on a similar bill sponsored by physician organizations. The lobbyists usually avoided discussing the facts of the bill. Instead, they kept repeating their mantras over and over: "This is a doctor protection act not a patient protection act."; "Get the government off our backs."; "Let the market regulate the system."; etc.

These lobbyists followed Ferguson's recommendations faithfully. But their arguments, although initially attractive, ultimately did not work. The lobbyists could never answer the crucial question posed by many of the legislators: "If managed care is doing such a good job, why are my constituents experiencing such problems and telling me such horror stories?" No matter how much public relations hype or how many favorable statistics from HMO-sponsored studies they quoted, the lobbyists simply could not answer that one question adequately. The legislators simply did not believe the lobbyists. They believed their own constituents. They listened to the voice of the people—*vox populi*. The passage of HB 335 represents a triumph of the republican form of government over the richest and most powerful interests in the state of Missouri.

As debate on the Senate version of HB 335 wound down, the business and insurance industries pulled out one last desperate stop. They marshaled their immense financial resources in recruiting "grass-roots" support to thwart passage of the bill. The United Auto Workers union enlisted their thousands of members to call legislators to oppose the bill. And Express Scripts, the huge mail order prescription company based in St. Louis, sent letters to its subscribers advising them to call their legislators to oppose the bill because their prescription costs would triple.

Anders also describes this type of grass-roots lobbying technique. He cites the experience of a Texas legislator who received many phone calls from his constituents opposing a managed care bill he was sponsoring. The legislator found that the phone calls were coming basically from an insurance company front organization—not from constituents who had made up their own minds independently. The angry legislator gave a speech in the legislature calling this type of activity "Astroturf" as opposed to grass-roots lobbying.

Legislators have shown themselves to be a lot smarter than the lobbyists gave them credit for. Many have experienced firsthand the problems of managed care. They are aware of Astroturf lobbying. And these tactics can backfire. For example, a supporter of HB 335 who received the letter from Express Scripts saying his prescription costs would triple told me he was outraged. He said he would try to have Express Scripts eliminated from bidding on his employer's prescription drug contract in the future.

By using misleading and emotional statements in their lobbying efforts, business and insurance interests only lower their own stature in the eyes of the public. A recent poll on the credibility of various businesses showed that only one industry—computers—was rated positively by over 50 percent of the responders. The public rated managed care second to last, just above the tobacco companies.

If the managed care industry and their business allies want to continue to attack the concerns of consumers and organized medicine with innuendo, half-truths and Astroturf lobbying as they have in the past, their public esteem will drop even further. They will not achieve their goals using phony propaganda. If the insurance and business interests want to sit down at the table and try to solve the problem of high medical costs in an open, fair, truthful and cooperative manner, the door will always be open.

❧

House Bill 335

We are very pleased to report that HB 335, the sweeping managed care reform bill, was given final approval, and the governor signed the bill on June 25, 1997.

- Gag clauses are banned;
- Managed care enrollees and prospective enrollees will be provided with explanations of a plan's benefits, preexisting condition limitations, limitations on

treatment options and referrals, any hidden out-of-pocket expenses, etc.;

- Managed care organizations will disclose how much of the premium dollar goes to administration and how much to actual patient care;
- Managed care organizations will provide a standardized grievance mechanism for patients;
- Managed care organizations will disclose any financial arrangements or contractual provisions that might limit or restrict the care a patient receives;
- Managed care organizations will maintain a network that is sufficient in numbers and types of providers to assure that all services will be accessible without unreasonable delay;
- Managed care medical directors will have to be licensed to practice medicine in Missouri;
- Managed care organizations will have to cover emergency services and cannot require preauthorization for those services;
- Managed care organizations cannot impose treatment limitations or financial requirements on coverage for mental health services if similar limitations or requirements are not likewise imposed on coverage for physical health services;
- If a patient's physician recommends a course of treatment and the insurance company denies coverage for that treatment, an appeals process would exist to reconsider the decision to deny;
- Deselected providers will be given an opportunity to appeal their termination; and
- Any insurer that offers a gatekeeper plan also must offer an open referral plan that allows enrollees to seek health care outside the managed care network.

Part Three

Hospitals Change Their Mission to Meet Threat of

Managed Care

The Transformation of America's Hospitals

Part One: The Hospitals and The Public
St. Louis Metropolitan Medicine
August 1999

Recently, a leading spokesperson for the American Hospital Association stated that a national Patients' Bill of Rights should not permit suits against managed care organizations. How can an institution claiming to be pro-patient come out against a strong Patients' Bill of Rights? An overwhelming majority of the American people as well as organized medicine support a strong Patients' Bill of Rights. They firmly believe that when an MCO makes medical decisions it should be held accountable through the courts just as physicians are. The AHA is taking the same position as the HMOs and large corporations.

It should come as no surprise that the AHA opposes a strong national Patients' Bill of Rights. When Missouri's HB 335, one of the strongest pro-patient laws in the country which permits suits against HMOs, was being debated in the Missouri Legislature two years ago, the Missouri Hospital Association initially opposed it. When its passage seemed assured, it took a neutral position.

For many years, the public trusted hospitals to be pro-patient. Hospitals were associated with religious organizations whose mission was to help the sick and the poor. There was cost shifting. Americans understood and accepted the fact that they paid higher insurance premiums to cover the health care costs of those who could not afford to pay. But times have changed. The public's trust of hospitals has waned. It is time to take a hard look at the causes of this transformation. It is time to look at who actually runs the hospitals and what their goals are.

Today, the executive committee of the board of directors runs the rest of the board and the hospital with an iron grip. The executive committee is composed mainly of corporate executives seething with anger over escalating health care costs, which lower their companies' bottom line. These executives intend to lower hospital costs by using the same methods they use to control costs in their businesses. They look to managed care as the way to accomplish this goal. They support managed care with a vengeance. Since they control the hospitals, the hospitals support managed care and oppose a strong Patients' Bill of Rights.

While the power of hospital boards has increased, hospital administrators have seen their authority diminish. Three decades ago, hospital administrators generally followed the directions of physicians and nurses. Two decades ago, hospital administrators donned power suits, took on the corporate titles of president and vice president, paid themselves handsome salaries, and developed their own power base. Over the past decade, with the onset of managed care, the executive committees of the board of directors have taken over the operation of hospitals, giving orders to administrators on major policies.

Even if hospital administrators wanted to improve quality or relations with doctors and nurses, if their efforts are perceived by the board as increasing costs, they are fired. Today, hospital CEOs come and go as through a revolving door. One might question whether hospital administration is an independent profession.

Everyone supports eliminating waste and promoting efficiency. However, recent hospital cost-saving programs have been overzealous and antagonized the public.

For example, both the quality and quantity of staffing of nursing divisions has decreased. Anecdotes, some amusing and some sad, abound. A psychiatric nurse told me that her hospital had hired new technicians from gambling boats because they were so "personable." At another hospital, a doctor made morning rounds on a sick patient being attended to by a person in a nurse's uniform. The doctor, recognizing the individual, asked, "Don't you work for housekeeping?" "I did until two months ago," responded the "nurse."

Obstetric nurses at one large local hospital went to the media because they felt so strongly that patient care was suffering because of nursing cutbacks. They enlisted the support of an obstetrician who agreed with them. The day after they spoke on the radio, the hospital fired two of the three nurses and the physician whose practice they had bought. They were unable to fire the one nurse who belonged to a union.

Because of patient care problems, nurses at another large local hospital are attempting to form a union. Unlike union management disputes in other industries, the major issue is not about wages and benefits. It is about the quality of care that patients receive.

Economists, business school professors, and antitrust lawyers sneer at doctors and nurses trying to form unions over so-called quality of care issues. They contend that professional issues are simply a smoke screen to cover up economic self-interest; they believe professional associations are nothing more than trade associations. In their one-dimensional view, man is pure and simply a *homo economicus.*

The public disagrees with these academic mavens. Quality issues do count for them. In California, after media publicity about patient care problems, Kaiser, the largest integrated health care delivery system in the country, had to make patient care concessions to the nursing profession. Now, the nurses must approve all staffing changes on nursing floors. In addition, the nurses significantly improved their financial position.

Local hospitals would do well to study the Kaiser experience. Unionization will eventually occur in St. Louis too if hospitals persist in staffing cutbacks. Cost-cutting efforts will prove counterproductive, causing costs to rise even higher than they were to begin with.

It is worth noting that while making staff cuts and jeopardizing the quality of patient care, hospital boards have not seen fit to exercise similar fiscal restraint in marketing expenses and capital expenditures. Nor have certain board members overlooked the opportunity to capitalize on their position of trust for personal gain.

Hospital networks are placing their logos everywhere from stadium domes to Big Mac Land at Busch Stadium. Whether advertising improves the bottom line of hospitals is unclear. What is clear is that it removes money that could be used for improving patient care.

Capital expenditures by hospitals also have increased. One local hospital is spending hundreds of millions of dollars in wrecking old buildings and putting up new buildings. There will be no net increase in the number of beds when the project is finished. Other hospitals have engaged in similar, albeit less ambitious projects. One might question whether such expensive projects siphon off money that could be used to provide health care for the tens of thousands of St. Louisans who have either insufficient or no health insurance and whose access to health care is limited.

To make matters even worse, many board members have personally profited from these hospital projects. Lawyers, accountants, bankers, stockbrokers, builders and others have seen business flow their way by virtue of their membership on the board. Crony capitalism is not just a way of life in emerging Third World economies. It is alive and well right here in the hospitals of our own city.

Membership on the board of directors of a not-for-profit hospital is a position of public trust. Members are supposed to sign a conflict of interest document which states that they will not profit personally from their positions on the board. Like all such documents which lack teeth, it has proven worthless. Whenever power is unchecked, it is abused. This lack of accountability has encouraged the unlimited avarice and hubris exhibited by certain board members.

Why should the average citizen be concerned about how boards run hospitals? The answer is that hospitals must be accountable to the public; if for no other reason than the fact that almost half of their revenue comes from the government through Medicare and Medicaid. It's our tax money that boards are playing with.

High health care costs are primarily a function of advancing technology and an aging population demanding unlimited services. Competition and increased efficiencies will have some modest effect, but they will not dramatically cut health care costs like they have the cost of television sets and computers.

If hospitals are to regain the confidence of the public and their pro-patient image, their boards must eliminate many of the hard-nosed methods of managed care. Managed care simply takes the caring and compassion out of the system for perhaps a minor, and often temporary, financial advantage. The solution, if there is one, to high health care costs and universal access will not come from managed care. It will come from the citizens of our country making difficult and painful decisions in a democratic way.

The   Transformation   of America's Hospitals

Part Two: The Hospitals and The Doctors
St. Louis Metropolitan Medicine
September 1999

Managed care has transformed American hospitals over the past decade as it has the practice of medicine. It is no secret that corporate America is driving managed care. In Minnesota and other states where managed care began, the large corporations were up front in stating that they were tired of paying double digit annual increases in health care bills for their employees. Taking matters into their own hands, they demanded that insurance companies do something about controlling health care costs. Thus, HMOs were born. Corporate America also has taken charge of America's hospitals through controlling the boards of directors and is initiating various cost-cutting strategies.

The relationship of hospitals to doctors is complex and ambivalent. On the one hand, hospitals want an ever-increasing market share. They want to attract as many physicians as possible to bring patients to their hospital. The smart hospitals know that it is the doctor, not the patient, who is their most important customer.

On the other hand, since large corporations are paying the hospital bills of many patients, they want to control utilization of resources and keep expenses down. If hospitals make physicians quasi employees and their membership on the staff contingent upon following certain practice guidelines, they can intimidate physicians into practicing medicine in a more "economically efficient" manner. This process is known as economic credentialing.

The major hospital strategy to improve market share has been to purchase the practices of physicians, mainly primary care physicians. The strategy to control physicians' practice patterns and engage in economic credentialing is through changing hospital bylaws. Both strategies are failing.

Almost a decade ago, the Health Care Advisory Board, a think tank which advises the 800 largest hospitals in the United States, recommended that in order to survive and guarantee a future revenue stream, hospitals should purchase physician practices. The goal is to "control physicians by employing them." By employing doctors, hospitals can ensure referrals, limit utilization and gain control over payers. The HCAB acknowledged that there are approaches other than employing physicians such as collaborating with them in an egalitarian manner or encouraging physicians to acquire and operate hospitals. The HCAB concluded that the latter option, "abdicating 100 percent control to physicians is too extreme a measure to stomach."

Note that the HCAB recommendation says nothing about the cost or quality of care that would result from purchasing physician practices. The strategy is strictly about ensuring hospital survival and retention of power in a period of health system reform.

In 1993, the St. Louis Metropolitan Medical Society convened a meeting with a number of hospital CEOs. At this meeting, I asked the CEOs if they intended to buy doctors' practices. Although one CEO admitted that his hospital had considered the matter, they unanimously said that their hospitals had no intention to purchase physician practices. Within two years, hospital networks were competing furiously with each other in a frenzy of purchasing primary care physician practices. Not one of those CEOs still heads a St. Louis hospital.

The HCAB thought that the strategy of buying practices might offend doctors. For once, I agreed with the HCAB. We were both wrong. With incomes plunging and the hassles of managed care increasing, physicians stood in line to accept salaries from hospitals which were often two to three times what they could earn in the marketplace. Many physicians never gave much thought to the possible ramifications of their decision to sell their practices. Their comments, if they made any, went something like the following: "Medicine is now a business." "One has to adjust to changing times." "This is a sound business decision."

Now the honeymoon is coming to an end. Hospitals are beginning to divest themselves of the practices which they had eagerly purchased a mere five or six years ago. The main reason for this change in strategy is, as usual, economic. All over the country, hospitals are losing between $80,000 and $100,000 per doctor per year. There was never any reason to believe that, in this era of shrinking reimbursement, hospitals could run offices more efficiently than physicians.

The hospital strategy of buying practices and developing large integrated systems hasn't worked. As one consultant put it "beyond the financial difficulties they (hospitals) are having in operating practices, they are not even meeting their objectives, such as protecting their referral base, increasing market share, and enhancing managed care contracting ... If you're losing money and not even meeting your goals, why do it?" The HCAB had given hospitals the wrong advice.

There is another reason for hospitals to divest themselves of practices. The IRS is cracking down on not-for-profit hospitals that pay above fair market value for practices. This kind of activity is known as inurement. Before 1997, the IRS could only eliminate the hospital's tax exemption. Now, it can fine hospitals. This is terrifying to both hospitals and their attorneys. Hospital attorneys have been frantically rewriting physicians' contracts or simply not renewing them.

Physicians, too, are becoming disillusioned with their employment by hospitals. At contract renewal time, the salaries offered are substantially lower than they had been with the first contract. There also are complaints by physicians about the number of patients they are required to see per day, lack of authority over staff, lack of control over coding and billing with its attendant legal risks, assignment of overhead, and loss of professional autonomy. Attorneys representing physicians now are reported to be as busy dissolving contracts between physicians and hospitals as they were a few years ago when physicians sold their practices. Many disgruntled doctors are retiring early.

While hospitals in St. Louis and elsewhere are losing millions of dollars yearly because of their purchase of physicians' practices, and while they also have been spending tens and even hundreds of millions of dollars on marketing and enormous capital expenditure programs, they are claiming the need to cut health care costs with an almost patriotic fervor. This is how they justify cutbacks in the quantity and quality of nursing care. And at the same time that they are investing in these unnecessary and extravagant spending programs which do not result in improved patient care or access, they are lobbying Congress and HCFA for more Medicare and Medicaid reimbursement!

Hospitals have employed a second strategy to control doctors. This strategy is based on control of the organized medical staff. From the beginning, the American Medical Association has seen this move by the hospitals coming. It has fought the hospital takeover of the medical staff tooth and nail. The entire thrust of the AMA Organized Medical Staff Section (formerly the Hospital Medical Staff Section) has been to ensure that the medical staff is a self-governing entity.

The self-governing authority of the medical staff is recognized by the Joint Commission for Accreditation of Health Care Organizations. Without accreditation by the JCAHO, a hospital may as well close shop. The self-governing authority of the medical staff also is recognized by state law.

Nevertheless, some prominent hospital attorneys see things differently. Some of their published "inflammatory and legally fallacious" statements intended to frighten doctors are pointed out in the AMA Board of Trustees Report 3 A-99.

"The medical staff of the hospital is no more separate than the nursing department."

"The notion that the hospital medical staff is something separate from the hospital itself ... is not only incorrect—it is legally dangerous."

"Physicians who may have thought that an independent medical staff was in their best interest will find themselves facing multimillion dollar antitrust and negligence suits as a result."

The differences in opinions between AMA and hospital attorneys are not just theoretical and of interest only to lawyers. Just recently, a large local hospital attempted to abrogate the independence of the organized medical staff by changing the bylaws. The hospital mandated that ballots were to be signed by physicians. The threat of reprisal against any physician voting against the bylaws change was obvious. The hospital medical staff sought and received legal assistance from the AMA. The hospital backed off, at least temporarily. The ruthlessness of the hospital in pursuing its goals is illustrated by its tactic of denying a secret ballot—one of the most basic and precious safeguards of the democratic process.

Why should physicians be very wary of or resist becoming employees of hospitals? And why should physicians insist on an independent self-governing medical staff? The answer is not difficult or complicated: It is so that physicians can act as the patient's advocate. This is the fundamental precept of the Hippocratic Oath.

When a physician becomes an employee of a hospital, his loyalty is divided between the patient and the employer who pays his salary. Early in this century, many companies employed doctors. The company doctors had divided loyalty. This in turn led to abuses. Because of these abuses, many states including Missouri passed laws which prohibit this practice known as the corporate practice of medicine. Now, history is repeating itself, and large corporations, in a misguided effort to control costs, are making the same mistake.

Recently, representatives of the SLMMS met with one of Missouri's most powerful and successful politicians who is currently running for high office. At the end of the meeting, he mentioned that during his travels across the state, people told him that doctors were the only group whom they trusted to represent their interests. They did not trust the hospitals, the HMOs, or their corporate employers to protect their interests.

By selling their practices to hospitals or allowing hospitals to control medical staff by laws and engage in economic credentialing, physicians run the risk of forfeiting the trust of their patients. That risk is just not worth taking.

The Transformation of America's Hospitals

Part Three: The Hospitals and Managed Care
St. Louis Metropolitan Medicine
October 1999

The two previous articles in this series have shown how hospitals have allied themselves with managed care by opposing strong patient protection laws, cutting back on nursing services and quality of care, and trying to control doctors' decision making. The third article will attempt to show how hospitals give preferential financial treatment to HMOs.

The reason for the hospitals' support of managed care is that the executive committees of the boards of directors are composed of leaders of the business community who strongly back managed care. As one board member put it to a colleague in a hostile, literally in-your-face way, "We like managed care!"

Hospitals have supported the concept of HMOs and given them steep discounts. At the same time, hospitals have been overcharging private and Medicare fee-for-service plans. Hospitals also have tried, although unsuccessfully, to become major players in managed care through the formation of integrated service networks.

One might expect hospitals and physicians to have similar opinions about managed care because managed care categorizes them both with the pejorative term "providers." Physicians often are critical of the policies of managed care; hospitals' criticisms, if they have any, are muted. These differences can be explained by the fact that doctors treat patients according to the Hippocratic Oath. The main goal of the corporate interests which now run hospitals is to cut costs.

Not only do hospitals support managed care, they have been one of the most important factors in causing the demise of fee-for-service medicine. Fee-for-service, according to managed care doctrine, is the fundamental cause of soaring medical costs. There is, however, little factual support for this doctrine. In the 1970s and 1980s, many studies showed that when doctors practiced *according to their best medical judgment* there was no significant difference in costs between HMOs and fee-for-service.

Almost a decade ago, hospitals began to offer steep discounts to HMOs. At a medical staff meeting of a local hospital, I asked the CEO the following question. "Why do you give discounts to HMOs and not indemnity insurance companies?" His answer: a wink and a "knowing" smile.

At that time, hospital care comprised about 40 percent of total health expenditures. Physician services constituted a little less than 20 percent. Some simple calculations show that if hospitals gave discounts to HMOs of 10 percent, 20 percent or 30 percent, total HMO costs could be reduced by 4 percent, 8 percent or 12 percent respectively. This discount alone would have provided enough cost savings to produce the death knell of indemnity insurance. Of course, there was another very important reason why insurance companies did not fight to preserve indemnity insurance. With HMOs, their share of the health care dollar and profitability increased tremendously.

In 1994, hospitals across the nation developed a health care system which would allow them to become the major player in health care. The Missouri Hospital Association proposal was called Independent Service Networks. These networks were to achieve cost savings through "vertical integration" and "economies of scale"—terms borrowed from economics textbooks. The governor of Missouri and many legislators supported this bill. Its passage seemed assured. (It should be noted that right up to the present, there have never been any studies showing that vertical integration in health care is cost effective.)

Many readers will remember that about 300 members of the St. Louis Metropolitan Medical Society went to the state capitol in Jefferson City to lobby legislators against passage of this bill. The bill did not pass in large part because of the efforts of physicians.

The St. Louis Business Health Coalition representing the largest corporations in the St. Louis metropolitan area (Civic Progress) also opposed ISNs—one of the few times that organized medicine and the SLBHC have agreed on anything. Of course the reasons that organized medicine and the SLBHC opposed ISNs were different. The SLBHC concluded that ISNs would constitute a monopoly of providers which would be unfair to business. Not that the SLBHC has anything against monopolies per se, it just prefers a different kind of monopoly—a monopoly of payers (monopsony). It is quite satisfied with the payer monopoly which, sorry to say, persists to this very day.

A story connected with ISNs illustrates how corporate America is firmly in command of hospitals. A hospital CEO gave a favorable presentation on ISNs to his hospitals' board of directors. The chairman of the SLBHC was a member of the hospital board and strongly opposed ISNs. The CEO got the message, quickly changed his mind, and never brought the matter up again.

Hospitals were not only instrumental in accelerating the change from indemnity health insurance to HMOs, they also have played a major role in driving beneficiaries from standard Medicare to Medicare HMOs. Families USA, a consumer health care research organization, published a report in 1996 on how hospitals were, in large part, responsible for the dramatic rise in the cost of Medigap premiums. In 1993, hospitals charged Medicare beneficiaries 217 percent of actual hospital outpatient costs. The steep increases in Medigap premiums caused by excessive hospital outpatient charges were a major factor in pushing seniors into switching to Medicare HMOs.

Medigap covers mainly Part B services which include doctor fees and hospital outpatient services. There was no rise in any area of physician Part B services. This was not the case for Part B hospital outpatient services where a "quirk" in Medicare reimbursement policy allowed the hospitals to charge whatever they wished to Medicare beneficiaries for their portion of outpatient costs. Medicare apparently forgot to cap these outpatient beneficiary charges as it has with inpatient charges by using diagnostic related groups.

Now Medicare is correcting this problem, but much damage already has been done. One has to wonder if hospitals operate according to a double standard. They give HMOs sponsored by private industry steep discounts while charging patients in standard fee-for-service Medicare whatever the traffic will bear.

Managed care organizations also are in part responsible for the financial crisis facing teaching hospitals because they have refused to contribute funds for teaching and research. MCOs benefit from the training of doctors. Without doctors, MCOs could not function, and without research, America's leadership in medical discoveries is jeopardized.

It is not surprising that MCOs refuse to pay their fair share to teaching hospitals and academic centers. Their fiduciary responsibility is to their shareholders not to teaching and research. The AMA and the academic community favor an "All Payer" system which includes Medicare and private health insurance in the financing of medical education. Legislation will be introduced in both Houses of Congress this year to provide an "All Payer System," but who knows when and if this bill will pass? Why do academic medical centers ask only the government and not managed care to bail them out of their financial crisis? By not requiring MCOs to contribute to graduate medical education, our nation allows its teaching hospitals to subsidize managed care. As usual, MCOs are getting a free ride.

However, the promise of managed care is fading. Health insurance premiums are again rising in some cases at double-digit levels for the coming year. Public opinion continues to rate managed care very low. And all the while, the number of uninsured continues to increase by about one million annually since the advent of managed care a decade ago. The hospitals have hitched their wagons to the managed care star. That star is falling.

The hospitals know that their image, like managed care's, is tarnished. Recently, some officers of SLMMS attended a meeting of the American Hospital Association. An AHA spokesperson admitted that the public's trust in hospitals has plummeted. In order to restore public confidence in hospitals, the AHA planned to embark on a public relations campaign to promote the "compassion" of nurses. The AHA brass must not read newspapers. If they did, they would learn that the nursing profession, fed up with hospital managed care policies, has successfully formed unions in St. Louis and across the nation in order to protect the quality of care that patients receive. The AHA spokesperson never mentioned the role of doctors. That is because, according to managed care gospel, doctors are pariahs—the root cause of high health care costs.

If the hospitals are serious about improving their image and regaining the confidence of the public, they are going to have to distance themselves from many of the practices of managed care. The likelihood of that happening is slim as long as the hospitals are under the firm control of the corporate backers of managed care.

The Transformation of America's Hospitals

Part Four: Unnecessary Hospital Construction Denies Care to the Uninsured
St. Louis Metropolitan Medicine
February 2000

Have you ever wondered how, in an era of fiscal austerity and excess bed capacity, hospitals are able to embark on enormous building programs? One large local hospital is in the process of undertaking a $320 million building project which, when completed, will add no additional beds. Another hospital network has just built a $40 million plush new office building. A third hospital network has just received approval to build a new $30 million women's hospital.

At the same time that these hospitals have embarked on extravagant building projects, the number of uninsured in the metropolitan area has grown to an estimated 210,000, of whom 71,000 reside in the city of St. Louis. The number of uninsured in the United States has increased to 43 million and is growing at a rate of over 1 million annually. Addressing the problem of the uninsured is one of the top priorities for the AMA and many specialty societies. Most political pundits think that it will be one of the most important issues in the 2000 national elections.

It is a sad commentary that the wealthiest country in the industrialized world has the highest number of persons without health insurance. No one seems to have a solution to this problem. In my opinion, if the money being spent on unnecessary and wasteful hospital building projects instead were used to provide health insurance to the uninsured, our society would be able to begin solving this serious problem.

Why do hospitals engage in extravagant building projects? There are several reasons.

The first reason is the unique way in which hospitals are financed. A book titled "The Hospital That Ate Chicago," published in 1979 by George Fisher, MD, describes the enormous tax subsidies which stimulate unnecessary construction. Fisher's analysis is complex. I will try to summarize his major points briefly. When hospitals borrow money for capital improvements the interest is reimbursed in cash by a third party which today is mainly the government. This essentially amounts to obtaining an interest free loan. Hospital construction is financed by tax-exempt bonds and when a hospital invests money, the interest is tax free. These tax breaks amount to a "staggering tax subsidy" to hospitals. These tax subsidies are a developer's dream—almost too good to be true. They entice hospitals into wasteful building projects.

I spoke to Dr. Fisher, an internist and an AMA delegate from Pennsylvania, at the recent AMA interim meeting. He believes 20 years later that his analysis is still correct. His book's conclusion is as valid today as it was in 1979. Fisher states, "You could give the whole $5 billion we spent on hospital construction last year to ... research as far as I'm concerned." Twenty years later, when hospital construction amounts to many billions more than in 1979, I would say "ditto" to Fisher's conclusion. However, I would propose using the saved money to help solve the problem of the uninsured rather than for research.

A second reason hospitals engage in extravagant building projects can be explained in psychological terms by those two basic human desires—power and money. Along with the generous tax subsidies described above, power and money (avarice) drive hospital boards of trustees, or more accurately, the executive committees of the boards, into these wasteful expenditures. Actual need for new buildings plays a minor role in my view.

As a contractor on one hospital project put it, the hospital builders are "like the pharaohs of ancient Egypt erecting pyramids, huge monuments to themselves." The decision makers at the highest level of hospital governance don't always have a focused purpose for their projects, changing their minds frequently during the building process. Often they don't consult the practicing physicians (or patients for that matter) for whom they are ostensibly building these monuments.

One surgeon told me that after a current building project is completed, the hospital will move his office 15 minutes away from the operating room. Whereas formerly, he could perform an operation, visit his office and see a few post-op patients between cases, now he has an additional half-hour tacked on. If a physician wants to visit a patient with complications who happens to be on the rehabilitation service of this hospital, he must walk two to three blocks—sometimes in bitter cold weather. And, if a sick rehab patient has to be transferred back to the acute care hospital, an ambulance is required. Newer isn't always better when practicing physicians are not consulted, but of course, the average doctor can't tell that to the board.

Money, or stated more clearly, the profit motive of individual board members, also drives these extravagant building projects. There is nothing wrong with the profit motive when it applies to private enterprise. But the board is in a position of public trust using public monies because almost half of hospital revenues come from taxpayer-funded programs — Medicare and Medicaid.

There is no reason for board members to profit financially by virtue of their position. It is an abuse of the public trust. Board members of all not-for-profit hospitals (which constitute about 3/4 of the hospitals in this area) are supposed to sign a conflict of interest statement which prevents them from personally profiting from their membership on the board. But, as with most rules which lack teeth, board members rarely pay attention to this document.

Recently, a local business publication reported that for the year 1998 a hospital paid one law firm over $450,000 and another law firm over $300,000 for professional services. Members of both law firms presently serve or have served in the past few years on the board of this hospital. When one looks down the list of the board members, one will find building contractors, accountants, bankers, investment brokers, etc., all of whom have profited personally from their board membership. And the bigger the deals, like huge construction projects, the more they profit.

This self dealing by hospital boards is not confined to St. Louis. It goes on throughout the country. Recently, the Allegheny system of hospitals centered in Pittsburgh with a net worth of over $2 billion (which is almost twice as large as the largest hospital network in the St. Louis area) went bankrupt. When the financial situation began to deteriorate, the board of directors of the hospital system did two things: it quadrupled its liability insurance and it paid back a large loan to the Mellon Bank. Directors of the

Mellon Bank served on the board of Allegheny. Is it proper for the Mellon Bank to lend money to a hospital system when its directors serve on the board of that hospital system? Is it proper when a hospital system has severe financial problems to pay off in full a creditor who sits on the board while other creditors may wait years for partial payment of debt?

The executive committees of the boards of not-for-profit hospitals represent the same corporate interests which back managed care. They firmly believe in the principle that free markets and competition will lower health care costs. That is, they believe in free markets and competition for everyone except themselves. They award many of the major "plums" of hospital business and construction to each other without competitive bids.

Board members, as captains of industry, proclaim their support for lower taxes and getting the "government off their backs and out of their lives." Yet, according to a recent article in *Modern Healthcare*, hospitals sent lobbyists to Washington who "successfully pressed lawmakers for relief from the Balanced Budget Act of 1997" which was supposed to restrain hospital construction. "Part of their strategy was to portray all the nation's hospitals as cash strapped institutions incapable of continuing existing services." The boards and hospital administrators are certainly not above accepting government-sponsored corporate welfare to fund their pet building projects even though "in principle" they oppose government spending and increased taxes.

The Poor and the Uninsured

How does hospital pyramid building affect health care to the poor and the uninsured? First it is important to understand how this group of persons presently obtains health care.

The Federal EMTALA "anti dumping" law compels all hospitals to admit seriously ill patients requiring hospitalization who present to the emergency room. These patients include the uninsured. Government vouchers reimburse much of the cost of these uninsured hospitalized patients.

The main problem for uninsured persons is in obtaining outpatient care for preventive medicine, chronic conditions, and acute ailments which do not require hospitalization. In St. Louis a system of clinics called ConnectCare has been set up to meet these needs. This system is facing an acute financial crisis. Funding has decreased because of both the phasing out of Regional Hospital funds and the termination of subsidies from the four major local hospital networks. According to a recent article in the *St. Louis Post Dispatch*, the funding shortfall amounts to about $11 million out of a total budget of $44 million needed to keep ConnectCare up and running.

Now back to the pyramid building. If the $400 million being used for unnecessary building projects in our area instead were invested at 6 percent interest, a return of about $24 million annually could be expected. If, in addition, the $150 to $300 million expected from the Blue Cross conversion from not-for-profit to for-profit settlement materializes, another $9 to $18 million annually would become available. These funds would be more than enough to cover shortfalls in outpatient care for all of the poor and uninsured in the St. Louis area in the foreseeable future. If there were a federal moratorium on all hospital construction, a similar scenario likely would play out in hundreds of cities across the nation where wasteful new hospital construction also is booming.

I propose the follow plan to make hospital boards accountable to the public, reduce unnecessary hospital construction, and better utilize our finite national resources to provide health care for the uninsured.

- Increase the size of hospital boards of directors to include patients and representatives of the general public. Since over half of the hospital revenue source flows from the government and public taxation, about half of the board should consist of such public members. They would assist in overseeing how the hospital spends money, look out for the public interest, and help prevent the board's executive committee from becoming a "good ol' boys club" as it is today.

- Hospitals should be regulated like public utilities because they use public money and are quasi monopolies. Presently, hospital boards are not accountable and this has led, as always, to abuse. Hospitals should be allowed to make a small profit and keep their charges to the public as low as possible.

- Develop civil penalties for profiting financially by virtue of one's membership on the board of directors of a hospital. Such penalties would put an end to self dealing by board members and help restrain hospitals from undertaking unnecessary building projects.

- Independent physicians who receive no compensation from the hospital should serve on hospital boards with full voting rights. Such physicians would provide objective professional input and also represent the interests of patients.

- Abolish the not-for-profit status of hospitals. All hospitals today including the so-called not-for-profit earn a profit. Both kinds of hospitals, as large corporations, function in pretty much the same manner.

Both kinds of hospitals render care to the indigent and uninsured because the EMTALA law requires all hospitals to care for all uninsured patients who present to emergency rooms. All hospitals should pay taxes.

- Abolish the tax breaks which stimulate unnecessary hospital construction. In the past, many U.S. hospitals were run by religious organizations, which perhaps needed tax subsidies for capital improvements and new construction. Today, hospitals are large profitable corporations. Basically, they are religious in name only. They no longer need tax subsidies.
- Declare a moratorium on all new hospital construction. If a definite need for a new hospital can be established, all stakeholders should be consulted. Current certificate of need laws need to be drastically revised.

The politicians say war is too important to leave to the generals. The financiers have said health care is too important to leave to the doctors. I submit that hospitals and health care are too important to leave to the financiers.

We, as a nation, are going to have to solve the problem of the uninsured, which is expected to reach 55 to 60 million in 2007. Currently, no one has even the slightest solution to this vexing problem. A moratorium on unnecessary and wasteful new hospital construction would constitute a first step in helping to address and solve this problem.

The Transformation of American Hospitals

Part Five: Academic Medical Centers, Professional Standards, and Managed Care
St. Louis Metropolitan Medicine
June 2000

As the teacher and guardian of professional standards, one would expect medical schools and academic medical centers to make a strong statement about the current changes in health care wrought by managed care. One hears academics individually complain about certain aspects of managed care, but the official position is silence.

The medical historian, Kenneth Ludmerer, MD, of Washington University School of Medicine, has duly noted this silence. In his recent book "Time to Heal," Ludmerer states: "What was notable for this book on medical education was not the degree to which the quality of care had deteriorated or improved under managed care but the absence of leadership of the nation's faculty in the debate over quality, even as managed care organizations were denying some of the most fundamental principles of medical professionalism. Traditionally, it had been academic medicine's responsibility to guard the nation's health by establishing and maintaining the standards of care."

" ... as the public became more and more anxious about the quality of care under managed care, little was heard from medical school leaders on the subject. Rather than challenge the more questionable practices of HMOs, most academic medical centers reacted to managed care as a *fait accompli*, and worked mainly to position their institutions to survive in the new marketplace—even adopting high physician 'productivity' . . . so they could better compete for managed care contracts. Academic medicine continued to speak of its unique altruistic and social mission. However, its actions suggested the primacy of self interest."

These harsh words criticizing the leadership of academic medical institutions are all the more significant since they come from a respected faculty member.

At recent grand rounds at an academic medical center, the speaker emphasized the importance of physicians' taking the time to explain to diabetic patients the importance of achieving good control of blood sugars in order to delay and prevent complications of the disease. Later on in his lecture, the speaker confessed: "I have six minutes to see a patient and in eighteen months that patient will no longer be in my panel."

What was the response of the medical school leadership attending the lecture to that statement? Silence. Deafening silence.

The governing council of a state medical association asked the dean of a medical school why it had accepted a teaching grant from Aetna Health Insurance Co. This was at a time when Aetna was imposing particularly onerous contracts on physicians in a number of states. The American Medical Association had publicly criticized Aetna's practices and had achieved some success in getting Aetna to back down. The dean's answer was "not to worry." He said that Johns Hopkins and a number of other prestigious medical schools also had accepted these grants. With government support for medical schools drying up, medical schools were forced to accept funding whatever the source.

In a historic role reversal, the governing council told the dean that the medical school should possess the moral authority to decline financial aid from a company so inimical to the interests of both physicians and patients. The survival of the medical school was not dependent on such grants.

In an article in the *New England Journal of Medicine* (Feb. 10, 2000), Jordan Cohen, MD, executive director of the Association of American Medical Colleges discusses why the AAMC opposes house staff unions. Cohen's stand on unions is understandable given his position. House staff unions will increase costs at academic health centers.

But then Cohen goes beyond the subject of just unions to address the topic of medical professionalism in general terms. He makes the following astonishing statement: "Nothing can protect patients as well as trustworthy physicians—no laws, no regulations, no patients' bill of rights, and certainly no union contract."

Cohen should know better than to downplay the importance of a strong patients' bill of rights. He should have a better grasp of history and law. Medicine, like any other profession, is part of a larger society. It is not practiced in a vacuum. There is a framework of rules and regulations, which govern the practice of medicine. These rules and regulations can permit or prevent physicians from acting as patient advocates. Certainly under the absolutist regimes existing in Germany and the Soviet Union during the last century, physicians could not practice as patient advocates. Nor can they under an absolutist corporate managed care system, which offers physicians financial incentives to deny care, and the prospect of being deselected if financial goals are not met.

Cohen then exhorts resident physicians to adhere to the principles "of the Hippocratic tradition." How better to promote the Hippocratic tradition than through a strong patients' bill of rights? The current patients' bill of rights passed by the U.S. House of Representatives and supported by the majority of Americans as well as organized medicine includes such Hippocratic Oath friendly rules as:

• allowing physicians to make medical decisions, not insurance companies;

• holding health plans accountable when they harm patients;

• allowing patients an independent, timely appeal if care is delayed or denied;

• ensuring adequate choice of treating physicians, including specialists.

The downplaying of the importance of laws, regulations, and a strong patients' bill of rights illustrates just how far medical schools have distanced themselves from engaging in meaningful discussions on professional standards in the era of managed care.

Academic medical centers have not just been silent about managed care. Many have embraced managed care. They have started faculty practice plans, which take capitated global risk contracts.

Recently, on the program "Frontline," national public television described one such plan that was profiled in the *New York Times*. The Beth Israel Deaconess Medical Center, affiliated with Harvard Medical School, lost $100 million in 1999. A primary care physician working for the plan is quoted as saying that he now must think constantly about expenses "every time I send a patient to the emergency room." If he spends too much, his income suffers. When a physician is asked what he thinks about a system where he must resist sending a patient to an out of network specialist even if it may benefit the patient, he responds, "I think it stinks."

The experience of many other faculty practice plans is similar. They are mired in red ink, declining practice standards, and low physician morale. Why have academic medical centers dedicated to teaching, research and quality medicine become involved in health care delivery systems so contrary to their professed values?

The answer, in my view, is straightforward—money. As pointed out by Ludmerer, over half of medical school funding now comes from clinical practice. The academic medical centers have sold their souls to managed care under the misguided notion that managed care can solve their financial problems. They have allowed financial types (some of whom have "MD" after their name) to usurp the traditional role of academic educators in determining how clinical medicine should be practiced.

By contrast, organized medicine, dismissed by many academics as nothing more than a trade association, has zealously fought for improved professional standards and patients' rights through legislation, the courts and the media.

Many academic physicians belong to organized medicine. The AMA has a section on education. There is a reference committee devoted entirely to medical education issues, which meets at both the annual and interim AMA meetings. Having served on this reference committee, I can testify that there is representation from all academic constituencies—students, residents, faculty and deans. The discussions are lively and partisan. Policy on medical education issues like all AMA policy is made democratically by popular vote on resolutions by the AMA House of Delegates.

Yet organized medicine and academic medical centers have taken different roads. In my view, it is organized medicine, not academic health centers, that has taken the high road. Perhaps when the present managed care era comes to an end and is replaced by a health care delivery system more attuned to the democratic values of our nation, academic medical centers will see the light and join organized medicine on that same high road. Whatever course academic medical centers take, future historians will duly record their actions.

The Transformation of American Hospitals

Part Six: New "Corporate" Hospitals Fail to Control Costs, Destroy Community Spirit and Support
St. Louis Metropolitan Medicine
January 2001

Free market economics has given Americans the highest standard of living in history. In order to control health costs large corporations, the insurance industry, antitrust lawyers, and business schools professors, with the support of the government, have banded together to apply free market economics to health care. Their efforts have produced managed care.

For hospitals this has meant the formation of competing networks and employing free market concepts such as advertising, market share, vertical integration, economy of scale and mergers.

A December 1999 report from the St. Louis Area Business Health Coalition, a research and policy making organization sponsored by the area's largest corporations, indicates that free market economics is not lowering hospital costs for corporate payers. The report concludes: "... significant cost efficiencies from hospital mergers (networks) have not as yet materialized." In fact the report raises concern that hospital systems have achieved such market concentration that they are shielded from competitive forces which in turn has led to higher prices.

Not only is free market economics failing to control

health care costs, it has produced a loss of community control of hospitals, eroded our democratic values, and distracted society from the important goal of achieving universal health coverage.

A half century ago, my father, Harry Gale, a businessman, served on the board of directors of the former Jewish Hospital for 17 years. At that time there was comparatively little public money available to hospitals. Physicians willingly spent many hours working in the clinics and attending on the medical and surgical floors without compensation. Professionals such as lawyers and accountants provided their services to the hospital gratis. Members of the board of directors did not financially profit by virtue of their position. The Auxiliary spent countless hours working to raise funds for the hospital. The community financially supported the hospital generously, as can be attested to by the bronze plaques with names of donors that can still be found in the corridors and on the doors of most patient rooms.

Members of the board were usually motivated by the traditional ethical value of charity and that quaint archaic concept, altruism, which, for all practical purposes, has disappeared from the lexicon. A similar culture prevailed across the country at most community not-for-profit hospitals. In that bygone era hospitals were truly not-for-profit community-based institutions unlike the corporate for-profit and so called not-for-profit hospitals we have today.

Today the public has little input into how hospitals are run or whether they should even continue to exist. Executives representing the interests of large corporations dominate the executive committees of hospital boards and make the major decisions. Their number one publicly acknowledged goal is to lower health care costs for the corporations on whose boards they also serve. Accepted societal goals of increasing access to health care for all Americans, considering the needs of the community served by the hospital, and improving quality are secondary.

In St. Louis, despite considerable community opposition, representatives of Civic Progress, an organization representing the largest area corporations, closed the last public hospital, Regional. A community leader and backer of Regional told me how saddened she and others were by the closing. She said that her community took great pride in Regional and considered it an excellent hospital. She then shrugged her shoulders and said that business leaders told her that Regional had to close for financial reasons and "for the good of society."

An example of the transformation of hospitals from community to corporate is the merger of Jewish Hospital with Barnes Hospital. Let me make it clear at the outset that the former Jewish Hospital, the former Barnes Hospital, and the merged Barnes-Jewish Hospital were and are excellent hospitals. That is not the issue.

Prior to the merger, Jewish Hospital had the best of both worlds—the efficiency and collegiality of a community hospital and the intellectual stimulation of a teaching hospital. The morale of the private and full-time physicians was high. The hospital always operated profitably with the exception of the year preceding the merger when, in a self-fulfilling prophesy, the administration deliberately began dismantling departments.

The board of directors of Jewish Hospital initially announced that there would be an affiliation not a merger between Barnes and Jewish hospitals. Then, contrary to their prior promises, the board and administration suddenly announced there was to be a merger. There was never any serious input in a democratic way from doctors, nurses, employees or even the community that supported the hospital.

In explaining the reasons for the merger the board and administration said, "It was for the good of society" — that economies of scale would accrue which would improve efficiencies and control costs.

As in the case of the closing of Regional, the board never cited any pilot studies or objective scientific evidence that would justify its decision that a merger would lower health care costs, or improve quality or efficiency. How can one even calculate cost savings? After the merger the majority of private physicians who formerly practiced at Jewish Hospital moved their practices to other hospitals mainly in the west central corridor.

There is little objective evidence that hospital mergers improve efficiency through economies of scale. Locally, St. Luke's and St. Anthony's Hospitals have separated from Unity, a large hospital network. The reasons given for the breakup by the attorneys for St. Anthony's as reported in the *St. Louis Post Dispatch* (June, 23, 2000) are instructive.

The Unity network "failed of its essential purpose in that the institutions ... did not realize the economies of scale or other efficiencies that had been anticipated at the time of the (merger) agreement in August 1995. As a result the formation of the network did not improve either the quality or the efficiency of the institutions' health care services, and in fact threatened to cause a deterioration in the quality and efficiency of such services." I suspect that these harsh words describing the St. Anthony's experience could be applied to many if not most hospital mergers.

What did the merger mean to the physicians,

employees, and the community that supported the former Jewish Hospital? One former benefactor perhaps summed up their responses best: "They destroyed history." The merger destroyed the tradition and spirit that animated community support for the hospital.

Hospital mergers are strictly top down decisions. That is the way big private corporations make decisions—not quasi-public institutions, which are in large part funded by the government and responsible to the community. Fifty years ago hospital boards had an unwritten social contract with the community they served. That social contract has been breached. Current hospital boards are accountable neither to the community or the government. Lack of accountability inevitably results in abuse of power. Even privately owned public utilities are scrutinized by regulatory agencies and hearings are held before mergers are approved.

The loss of public support for hospitals is understandable. Except for research or educational funds, why would public spirited philanthropic citizens seriously consider donating time, effort or money to a so-called not-for-profit community hospital which:

- would pay the CEO of the system to which the hospital belonged over a million dollars per year and then pay that individual half of that salary for five years or life after he or she left the system either voluntarily or involuntarily?

- would belong to a network which simply adds another layer of bureaucracy to the hospital's own bureaucracy employing hundreds of persons and adding tens of millions of dollars of costs in increased salaries and benefits?

- would spend $40 to $70 million for a building (since

sold) with posh offices, waterfalls and fountains just to house the network's bureaucracy?

- belongs to a network that would purchase physician practices and lose $80,000 to $110,000 per year per doctor or over $20,000,000 per year?
- belongs to a network that spends millions of dollars on marketing, including placing logos and huge signs at professional sports stadiums in order to increase "market share"?
- belongs to a network that sponsors an HMO which loses millions of dollars per year?
- would engage in unnecessary building projects that cost hundreds of millions of dollars and which use massive tax breaks that the ordinary taxpayer must subsidize?
- allow certain members of the board of directors to obtain financial windfalls by virtue of their membership on the board?
- would cut back nursing care to patients while supporting a bloated administrative bureaucracy?
- tries to impose bylaws (Horty Springer) on the medical staff that economically credentials physicians, makes physicians quasi employees of the hospital, and prevents them from acting as patient advocates?

All of these unnecessary changes and expenditures are being made while the number of uninsured in our nation has increased from 33 to 43 million during the past decade. They are being made while we physicians have to rummage through our medicine closets for sample drugs as stopgap treatment for our Medicare patients who cannot afford the medication necessary for the treatment of their chronic diseases. These extravagant and wasteful hospital expenditures are absurd. Every dollar spent on unnecessary salaries, buildings and advertising is a dollar less spent on patient care. The current corporate takeover of hospitals primarily benefits MBAs, marketers, contractors and financiers, not the public.

Is there a future for community not-for-profit hospitals? Are the conditions that gave rise to community hospitals now obsolete? Should they lose their tax-free status? If community hospitals are run, as they are today, in an authoritarian manner primarily to serve the financial interests of large corporations, then it is probably better to drop all pretense and allow them to become for-profit hospitals like the chains. If they are to remain community institutions and retain their tax free, not-for-profit status, they are going to have to operate in a more democratic way that allows input and some control from all stakeholders including physicians, nurses and the community. It is important to remember that hospitals belong in large part to the public since over half of their funding is tax supported.

It has been said that economists know the price of everything and the value of nothing. The current transformation of American hospitals has not benefited the public in either lowering price or enhancing value. By their own analysis the corporate takeover of hospitals is not reducing health care costs. In addition it is having the unintended effect of helping to destroy the values and bonds that hold a democratic society together.

The Transformation of American Hospitals

Part Seven: So Called "Free Market" Fails, A New Strategy with More Accountability is Needed
St. Louis Metropolitan Medicine
October 2001

Over the past decade, in a misguided and failed effort to cut costs, big business has recast hospitals in its own image. It has imposed a new god, "free market" economics, onto health care. This new religion was supposed to transform not-for-profit public service hospitals into hard-nosed bottom line competing corporations. Hospitals under the managed care theory were to become the flip side of HMOs. Competing hospital systems would constitute the provider side while competing HMOs were to be the payer side in this brave new world.

Perhaps the corporate community had good intentions when it scrapped the former hospital system that was at least nominally under the control of religious institutions and where the insurance premiums of those who could afford them subsidized those who could not. Perhaps the demise of this system was inevitable. However its replacement with a free market system, which is not truly a free market system, has been a dismal failure. In attempting to emulate business practices that work in the private sector, hospitals have squandered billions of dollars that could have been used for patient care where it is desperately needed.

Eighty-five percent of the hospitals in the United States are nonprofit, and 45 percent of hospitals are in integrated systems. These are the hospitals that have engaged in the most egregious practices that waste precious resources. Hospital systems have spent enormous sums of money on marketing, information systems and administrative salaries. They continue to lose staggering sums on vertical integration (the purchasing of doctors' practices and owning HMOs) and horizontal integration (hospital mergers) in a quixotic quest to improve efficiency by achieving economy of scale. Finally they have spent literally billions of dollars on unnecessary building projects and capital improvements supposedly to attract patients.

We will briefly examine each of these practices.

Is hospital marketing directly to the public really worthwhile? How often do patients ask doctors to send them to a hospital system touted on a traffic helicopter or because they saw Mark McGwire hit a home run over a large expensive sign at Busch Stadium? The answer is obvious — never. Doctors are the customers of hospitals not patients. Patients in time of medical crises go to hospitals that their trusted doctor recommends. Hospitals would do far more to improve their image by taking the money that they spend on marketing to improve patient care.

Hospital administrative costs are spiraling. According to one expert who analyzed data from the American Hospital Association, the growth in staff to patient ratio has increased on the administrative not the clinical side "reflecting increased staffing for marketing, public relations, and information technology." (This insight comes as no surprise to most doctors.) The expert admonishes hospitals: "If you reduce your length of stay but you don't reduce your workforce, productivity declines."

Over the past decade health care reformers from America's business schools preached the virtues of "seamless" integrated hospital systems. Several years ago at an AMA meeting I heard one young MBA sermonize with evangelical fervor about the dawn of a new utopian health care millennium. The reformers' sweet siren song convinced hospital trustees, desperate for a quick fix for rising health care costs, to implement their unsubstantiated theories. This costly mistake is largely responsible for the current sorry state of affairs in the hospital industry. Harvard Business School Professor Regina Herzlinger in her book "Market Driven Health Care" convincingly refutes the reformers' theories by marshalling studies that conclusively demonstrate that vertical integration does not improve efficiency and drives up hospital costs.

All three local not-for-profit systems have lost hundreds of millions of dollars employing physicians. Across the country hospitals lose on average $100,000 per year per doctor. Although some systems are beginning to eliminate physician practices, mainly in primary care, many hospitals continue to own and even purchase new practices. One local hospital system currently owns 140 physician practices losing approximately $14 million per year. So why do hospitals vertically integrate by buying physician practices and owning HMOs, since they are not efficient and increase rather than decrease costs? Answer: To obtain referrals to the hospital. The more basic question of who ultimately pays for these hospital losses will be addressed later.

Previous articles in this series have recounted the enormous sums hospitals spend for new building projects. In the St. Louis metropolitan area alone there is currently over a billion dollars being spent or projected for new brick and mortar projects. Despite hospital closings in inner cities and rural areas, and despite severe fiscal restraints on the most important hospital function, patient care, hospitals all across the nation are on a building binge. In most cases older facilities were perfectly adequate and simply required modernizing.

The theory that a free market system as exists in the private sector would work in health care where the vast majority of hospitals are still "nonprofit" is fundamentally flawed. First of all the term nonprofit in a profit-driven free market is an oxymoron. More importantly, when hospital systems go into debt what do they do? They ask their rich Uncle Sam (the taxpayer) to bail them out.

How is this a free market system? Would the public allow the government to bail out General Motors, Microsoft, or any other large corporation if it lost money because of fiscal mismanagement? A free market exists in health care in name only. Adam Smith would likely turn over in his grave if he learned how his theories have been misapplied.

After the balanced budget act of 1997 was passed, many hospitals experienced financial difficulties. They then successfully lobbied the government and received billions more in reimbursement. Now the nonprofit hospital systems are again taking their tin cup to the government, begging for more money. Their lobbying campaign is linked to the nursing shortage. The hospitals claim they need extra money to hire and train more nurses when actually they need an additional government handout because of extravagant, unnecessary spending on items that do not improve patient care.

The Need for More Accountability

The lobbyist for nonprofit hospital systems might find it more difficult this time convincing Congress that they need more money. True, their current profit margins are small, but under the same reimbursement system and a similar patient mix, most of the investor-owned hospital chains are quite profitable. I am not trying to make a case in support of for profit hospital chains. But I am trying to make the case for more accountability for nonprofit health systems, an accountability that is virtually nonexistent.

I am not the only one who thinks this way. The November-December 2000 issue of *Health Affairs*, a respected health economics journal, published four articles that called for more accountability and more public service from nonprofit hospitals. The authors conclude that the public is not getting its money's worth from nonprofits. The specter of hospital systems losing their tax-exempt status if the public becomes sufficiently disenchanted is a distinct possibility. The corporate takeover of nonprofit hospitals has undermined the social compact with the public that formerly existed and which was the original basis for their being granted tax-exempt status.

The responsibility for the transformation of American nonprofit hospitals into competing corporate systems with the ensuing massive losses of public monies lies squarely with their governing boards. The governing boards of the nonprofit hospital systems are controlled by CEOs of large corporations, the same CEOs who ardently support HMOs and managed care as a means of lowering health care costs. These CEOs run the hospitals like they run their corporations with absolute top-down power. They shun input from medical staff, nurses, and the general public. They have never been held accountable for their actions. It is ironic that their transformation of American hospitals has not produced the anticipated monetary savings for their companies.

How is accountability to be achieved? There is a strategy. It is as old as our nation. It's called democracy. Why not hold public elections for at least one-half of the membership of the board of directors of nonprofit hospitals? Such elections would be similar to the way school board members are elected. After all, almost one-half of the reimbursement of hospitals comes from Medicare and Medicaid, which are completely taxpayer funded. And huge public subsidies through tax-exempt bonds enable hospital systems to obtain interest-free loans for their monumental building projects.

When the St. Louis Cardinals wanted to build a new $350 million baseball stadium (which incidentally is expected to cost less than the estimates for each of the building projects of two local hospital systems), they first had to obtain approval from elected officials in the state legislature and the governor. When shopping center developers use tax subsidies (tax increment financing or tifs) they must first obtain approval from elected officials — aldermen and the mayor of the local community. Hospital systems have no such accountability in their use of public monies and tax subsidies. They submit their projects to a state appointed Certificate of Need Committee that has basically been a rubber stamp. Publicly elected trustees representing the public interest would demand public accountability. They could demand that hospitals open their books for inspection.

Public election of hospital trustees may sound preposterous. It is certain to meet fierce resistance from the current boards of nonprofit hospital systems whose absolute power would be threatened. Surprisingly this approach to hospital governance is neither preposterous nor novel. It is already in existence in certain areas of the country. In fact board members are publicly elected at a mid-Missouri hospital that is affiliated with one of the local hospital systems.

Contrary to the opinion of the free market health care reformers, there is no one ideal utopian solution to health care problems that will satisfy everyone. Nor can any program like the Clinton plan or managed care be imposed on the American people against their will. Any acceptable solution to health care problems will entail painful compromises for all Americans. The only way to reach compromise is through the democratic process. It's time to take inventory of past failures, rekindle public discussion on important health care issues, and try new approaches.

The Transformation of American Hospitals

Part Eight: Message for Hospitals From the Enron Collapse: "Open Your Books"
St. Louis Metropolitan Medicine
April 2002

The genius of our American democracy is the creation of a constitution with checks and balances. The founders knew, in the words of James Madison, that men were not angels. For a democratic government to work, individuals have to be held accountable.

Likewise the genius of the capitalist free market system is accountability. In order for free markets to work there must be full disclosure of all financial information to investors. Hubris, greed and conflicts of interest were not the direct cause of Enron's bankruptcy. These behaviors are universal. Lack of full financial disclosure and accountability ultimately doomed Enron.

There is a message to American hospitals from the demise of Enron. A recent editorial in *Modern Health Care* (Feb. 4, 2002), a journal devoted primarily to hospital issues, points to the need for nonprofit hospitals in the wake of Enron to open their books to the public. Most American hospitals are still nonprofit and are not subject to "the federally mandated disclosure requirements and accounting standards of public companies."

There have been two high profile failures of nonprofit hospital systems that are similar to Enron. In both of these cases the hospital systems gave incomplete financial information to the public.

In 1998 the Allegheny Health, Education and Research Foundation declared bankruptcy. Allegheny, a huge nonprofit 14-hospital Pittsburgh based health system, failed basically because it did not disclose sufficient financial data to its creditors. The actions of Allegheny were so egregious that four former executives and three former auditors are to be criminally tried in Federal Court for securities fraud.

The second case is that of Allina, a nonprofit hospital system in Minnesota. The integration of Allina's 16 hospitals and 47 clinics with its health plan in 1994 was trumpeted with great fanfare as a future model for all U.S. health care delivery systems. Now, after an 18-month financial audit, the Minnesota attorney general rebuked and penalized Allina for excessive spending for corporate travel and entertainment, overpayment and lax oversight of consultants, and conflicts of interest between hospital and health care divisions. State investigators found that Allina health care plan spent 18.7 percent of its revenues on administration, almost twice as much as the 9.9 percent it reported to the Minnesota Department of Health. Allina also has offered to pay $16 million to settle a federal investigation.

Simply put, Allina administrators enriched themselves at the expense of the public. From now on Allina is required to publicly disclose all administrative spending. If this requirement had been in place previously, the Allina debacle would not have occurred.

The Allegheny and Allina cases illustrate a fundamental flaw in the reporting of financial data by nonprofit hospital systems. Nonprofit hospital systems are able to conceal from the public crucial financial information.

Let's take a local example. A hospital in Northwest County recently requested and received $200,000 from the St. Louis County Council to help underwrite the cost of a trauma center. The hospital is seeking up to a million dollars for this project. The necessity of having a trauma center at this location is undeniable. It also is undeniable that the integrated health system to which the hospital belongs has millions of dollars available to fully fund this project if it simply managed its finances properly.

This hospital system, just like the other two hospital systems in the St. Louis metropolitan area, loses millions of dollars annually on the primary care practices it owns. It spends millions of dollars on marketing and administrative salaries and tens of millions of dollars on questionable construction projects. If a hospital system requests a public handout then the public has a right to know exactly how its hard-earned tax dollars are being spent.

Now the area's largest employers have entered the fray and are seeking detailed financial data from hospitals in order to lower health care costs. In fact, a bill introduced in the Missouri Legislature by the St. Louis Business Health Coalition, which represents the largest employers in the St. Louis area, would require hospitals to open all of their financial records to the public. Under current law hospitals are required to report detailed financial data to the Missouri Department of Health. The Department uses the data to produce consumer guides and other studies for public consumption, but the detailed financial data is not made public. It should come as no surprise that the Missouri Hospital Association vehemently opposes this bill.

Increased hospital costs have fueled large employers' demands for more hospital financial accountability.

Hospital costs have now surpassed pharmaceuticals as the fastest growing source of increased health care spending.

In an ironic twist, it is the employers themselves who are responsible for the creation of integrated systems and increased hospital costs. Over the past decade self-anointed "experts" from the business world swept across the country meeting with hospital boards and proclaiming the improved efficiency and cost savings that would result by installing competing integrated systems. Their rosy predictions have never been fulfilled. In fact just the opposite has occurred. The boards that gave their support and blessings to integrated hospital systems have created a Frankenstein monster that has spun out of control and is in the process of devouring them.

What is the solution to this problem? The first solution would be to simply jettison the entire concept of integrated hospital systems. In this vein, it is worth quoting the astonishing statement of Allina's new chair, John Morrison.

A chastened and remorseful Morrison, obviously stung by the disgraceful behavior of his predecessors, is refreshingly frank: "If the parent company (Allina) doesn't provide...(value added service) then you have to put the money and the power...with the doctors and the nurses. We're not here to perpetuate the life styles of executives; we're here to perpetuate the delivery of good health care."

Let's take a closer look at the first part of Morrison's statement: "If the parent company doesn't provide 'value added service'." If hospitals disclosed full financial data, the public would soon discover that integrated hospital systems provide no value added service and have instead become enormous money losing cost centers. For example, in St. Louis administrative costs of a hospital network (including information systems) can run as high as $50 or $60 million per year; executive salaries can top $1 million. One network's administrative headquarters equipped with fountains, waterfalls, and brooks rivaling those of the palace of Versailles cost between $50 and $70 million.

The public might be shocked to discover how hospital systems lose tens of millions of dollars yearly in ownership of unprofitable managed care plans and physician primary care practices. The public also might be surprised to find out how it subsidizes extravagant and often unnecessary building projects by granting hospitals the right to issue tax-free bonds. The huge sums spent on these wasteful projects and unnecessary administrative perks could be better spent on patient care where increased funding is desperately needed.

The second part of Morrison's statement "then you have to put the money and the power with the doctors and nurses," coming as it does from a hospital system executive, is truly earth shaking. Morrison is essentially recommending that we return to the way hospitals were run before the MBAs took charge. We have now come full circle because of the admitted failures of the present system.

To Morrison's fellow hospital system executives his statements constitute heresy. In fact some might even think that he must have lost his mind—perhaps as a result of a post-traumatic stress disorder induced by the collapse of Allina. So, despite Morrison's candid confession, I would not recommend holding one's breath waiting for hospital system administrators to voluntarily give up their power and income.

What will change hospital behavior? The answer is the same as it is for Enron—full disclosure of financial information. Publicly owned companies have to meet this requirement. So should not-for-profit hospitals. The taxpayer through Medicare and Medicaid publicly finances approximately almost half of all hospital revenue. And now employers who finance the other half of hospitals' revenue also are clamoring for more financial data.

It's time to let the sun shine in. It's time to enact laws requiring hospitals to report detailed financial information. After all, accountability is as fundamental to our capitalistic free market system as it is to our democracy.

The Transformation of American Hospitals

Part Nine: Economics not Efficiency Underlies the Formation of Hospital Networks
St. Louis Metropolitan Medicine
September 2002

Over the past decade American hospitals engaged in "merger mania." These networks were supposed to emulate the large corporate conglomerates of the private sector and through competition lower health care costs. In the words of the governing boards and administrators of hospitals, "economies of scale" achieved by mergers would result in greater efficiency and cost savings. The public believed these words. After all, they came from some of the most respected members of the community.

A new book titled "Health Networks: Can They Be the Solution?" forever lays to rest the theory that hospital networks cut costs. The main purpose of hospital networks, according to author Thomas P. Weil, is the formation of oligopolies to "enhance bargaining ability when negotiating with managed care networks." Networks enable hospitals to "increase market penetration, and improve bottom line performance."

That hospital systems seek oligopoly status and the elimination of competition was amply demonstrated in the recent session of the Missouri legislature. Hospitals and their business allies introduced a bill that required Certificate of Need approval for independent freestanding surgery, cardiac catheterization, and imaging centers, etc., but would exempt hospitals. This brazen bill, had it been enacted, would have restricted competition and created an unfair advantage for hospitals no matter how inefficient they were.

Weil marshals evidence demonstrating that hospital mergers (horizontal integration) do not decrease costs and that freestanding independent hospitals are as efficient as merged hospitals. His analysis also confirms that vertical integration (the ownership of physician practices and managed care plans) loses money and recommends that hospital networks rid themselves of these monetary albatrosses.

Weil also deplores the lack of public disclosure of financial information by not-for-profit hospitals—a requirement incidentally that for-profit hospitals must meet as mandated by the Security Exchange Commission. He also decries the swollen and ever-increasing administrative costs of hospitals and the entire U.S. health care system.

Weil is uniquely qualified to analyze hospital networks. After working for a number of years as a tenured college professor and director of a graduate program, he changed careers to become, for the past two decades, a full-time hospital consultant. His knowledge of hospital networks is therefore balanced as it comes from both the perspective of a respected academic scholar and as a hands-on insider who advised hospitals during their conversion to networks. In an understated aside, Weil says that his views were and still are "not always consistent with conventional wisdom."

If one accepts Weil's basic conclusion that the main purpose of networks is the formation of oligopolies, one can easily understand why health care costs are rising out of sight. Hospital networks were formed not to improve efficiency, as the public was led to believe, but out of fear of managed care. Hospital networks are simply the other side of the managed care coin.

While pretending to favor a competitive health care system, hospitals actually were terrified that managed care would dictate financial concessions that would drive down their bottom line and even put them out of business. So they formed network oligopolies. Oligopolies and monopolies by definition increase prices to consumers. This explains why at the present time hospitals have surpassed pharmaceuticals as the most rapidly escalating drivers of health care costs (*Health Affairs*, Vol. 20, Number 6, 2001). And lest we forget, hospital expenditures devour almost 40 percent of the health care dollar, by far the largest item in our health care budget.

The formation of hospital networks and managed care in general is based on the erroneous assumption that so-called free market principles can be applied to health care. Free market capitalism does provide market discipline for inefficiency. If a business fails to be profitable, its market value sinks and bankruptcy may ensue. Witness the current tanking of the stock market and wave of corporate bankruptcies.

Although hospital networks like to think themselves free market players, they aren't. Eighty-five percent of hospitals are not-for-profit; so right off the bat, it is an oxymoron for them to call themselves "free market" competitors. Secondly, when they encounter financial difficulties, they always run to the government asking for a bailout. Through effective lobbying, hospitals were able to restore $50 billion of the $112 billion cut intended by Congress in the balanced budget act of 1997. Is this behavior consistent with a free market?

The failure of hospital networks to cut health care costs leads to some important questions: How did hospital networks come about? Could their formation have been prevented? And now that networks are firmly in place, what is the solution to spiraling hospital costs?

Weil devotes only one paragraph in his 344-page book to explain how hospital networks came about. But it is an extremely enlightening paragraph and right on the mark. It describes to a "T" what happened in boardrooms as hospital trustees grabbed power from the public and physicians.

"... How you integrate the community's various publics in the merger negotiations can become ... a contentious issue because the public and the medical staff believe that an acute care hospital ... is a community resource and its future destiny should be shaped by *representatives of its many interested parties*;" (italics mine). On the other hand "a not-for-profit governing board (most often made up of community leaders and a few key physicians) usually suggests that the topic of merger is too complicated for public discussion; the negotiations are ... more effectively handled behind closed doors; and the decision ... to merge should be left to the 'experts.' This 'closed door approach' might be perceived as, or in fact be, most beneficial to the professional and personal interests of those 'in power.'"

So there you have it. The formation of hospital networks was undertaken behind closed doors in secret without input from the public or physicians. This power grab by an elitist group of "honorable men" serving on hospital boards all across the nation represents a cynical disregard or, more aptly put, contempt for the democratic process.

They were going to run their hospitals as they saw fit, just like they run their large corporations. They were going to control skyrocketing health care costs without any input from the public or from physicians (whom they blamed for increased employer health care costs).

Now it is obvious that their experiment with hospital networks is a failure. I recently attended a meeting of benefits managers of some of the largest corporations in the metropolitan area. These managers were so frustrated by rising employee health care costs that several mentioned that employers could no longer afford giving health benefits to employees and that the only solution might be a single payer system. The latter comment was a bit surprising, given the source.

I asked one of the attendees at this meeting why their bosses, the CEOs of large corporations who also sit on the boards that run the networks, allow hospitals to engage in spending binges. No answer was forthcoming. The CEOs, a.k.a. hospital board members, are sabotaging their own companies' employee health plans by approving expenditures that raise health care costs. And then they complain that they can't afford health insurance for their employees!

Could the formation of hospital network oligopolies have been prevented? I think so. Had the public debated the pros and cons of hospital networks, we might have seen a different outcome. Whatever one thinks of the Clinton Health Care Plan, to its credit, it was submitted for approval in a democratic way to the American people. The media and public debated and discussed it extensively. And finally, in a democratic way, the American people rejected it.

On the other hand, hospital networks, just like the

HMOs that preceded them, were rammed down the throats of the American public without public debate or approval. The HMOs have paid dearly for this lack of public support and input. The public now holds them in such low esteem, in fact, that they rank just above the tobacco companies in polls. Hospital networks run the same risk once consumers and taxpayers figure out that hospital networks are oligopolies that raise prices.

What is the solution to out of control spiraling hospital costs? Weil predicts that when there is a turndown in the economy the public will demand control of hospital spending. He predicts that the present hospital networks will survive, but they will be regulated like other monopolies such as public utilities. Weil admits, however, that public utility commissions usually become captives of the industries they are supposed to regulate. My own view is that a far better system of regulating hospitals would be to have at least one half of the boards of not-for-profit hospitals elected by the public. Admittedly, democracy is slow, messy and often indecisive. But it has a proven history of success. Consumers and taxpayers would have been better served by moving slowly and incrementally than by being rushed into what we have now, a health care system dominated by spendthrift, unaccountable, and unregulated hospital networks.

Weil has performed a great public service by exposing hospital networks as oligopolies. To the question posed in the title of his book, "Health Networks: Can They Be the Solution?" his answer is simply, "Unfortunately, no." The public may not read this scholarly book, but its conclusions should be widely disseminated to every citizen, especially legislators, when the hospitals come calling, asking for another handout.

Part Four

Managed Care is a Failure

America's Best Kept Secret: Managed Care is a Failure

St. Louis Metropolitan Medicine
February 2003

A decade ago, health care costs were rising annually at double-digit rates, and the number of uninsured had risen to 31 million. Government, business and the public were becoming alarmed. Two health care plans were being touted to the American people as the solution to both rising health care costs and the increase in the number of the uninsured. Both were backed by so-called experts from government, academia and business. One was called the Clinton health plan. The other was called managed care. For a variety of reasons, the public rejected the Clinton health plan. Managed care probably would have met the same fate had the public been allowed to voice its opinion.

Because our health care system is employer based, corporate CEOs and large insurance companies combined to force managed care on our nation. We tend to forget that since the end of World War II, employers have given employees health benefits in lieu of wages. Because employers do not pay payroll taxes on employee health benefits, they save billions of dollars annually. Since it is their wages that are being spent, employees should have had input into the kind of health care they will receive. The imposition of an untried and unproven system, managed care, on employees and the public without their prior input or approval is a breakdown of the democratic process and an abuse of power.

Now, 10 years later, it is clear that managed care is a failure. Health care costs continue to rise annually at double-digit rates, and the number of uninsured has risen to 41 million. The number of uninsured would have risen to 44 million had Congress not enacted the Children Health Insurance Program. And, although we are in the midst of a health care crisis, managed care just keeps merrily rolling along as if nothing is wrong.

In order to understand why and how managed care failed it is necessary to examine the roles of all the major players.

The Government

In the mid-1970s, two major court decisions paved the way for the managed care takeover of medicine. In the Goldfarb decision, the U.S. Supreme Court removed all professions including medicine from antitrust exemption. The theory behind the court's decision was that professions used antitrust exemption to restrain trade and fix prices.

Following the Goldfarb decision, the Federal Trade Commission successfully sued the American Medical Association (AMA vs. FTC) over a section in its "Principles of Medical Ethics." The court compelled the AMA to remove a section that stated, "a physician should not dispose of his services under ... conditions which ... tend to interfere with or impair ... his medical judgment ... or tend to cause a deterioration of the quality of medical care." Most Americans expect physicians as a matter of course to practice in accordance with this principle, which is virtually identical to the Hippocratic Oath.

The court took a different view. It interpreted this

section as prohibiting doctors from working for HMOs. One must understand that in the 1970s, elitist policy makers, judges and antitrust attorneys held that "free market economics" and HMOs were the solution to rising medical costs. They also believed that doctors opposed HMOs for pocketbook not ethical reasons. Now, history has proved the experts wrong. But the two court decisions stand and have had the net effect of lowering the standards of medical practice without the redeeming effect of lowering health care costs.

Large Corporations

Large corporations were the driving force behind the managed care revolution. Corporate CEOs were seething with anger over rising health care costs for their employees. They believed that by bringing the same free market concepts to health care that had worked so well in the private sector, costs could be controlled. Politicians of all stripes also hopped on the bandwagon. They, too, thought that managed care would solve the fiscal problems they faced with Medicaid and Medicare.

Over the past several years, it is apparent to all that the managed care bubble has burst. Free market concepts as applied by managed care don't work in health care for the following reasons.

- A free market cannot operate when third parties pay the bill. An example: American hospitals have lost billions of dollars in their financially disastrous ventures of purchasing physician practices and starting their own HMOs. A truly free market would have disciplined these hospitals by forcing them into bankruptcy. Instead, the hospitals ask the government for a bailout explaining that their poor business judgment is just part of the normal cost of doing business. When Chrysler asked the government for a bailout for its poor business decisions, some years back, it caused a public furor.

- Free markets, through the use of advertising, exert inflationary pressures on health care expenses by inducing consumers to use services and products whether they need them or not. Direct advertising to consumers by pharmaceutical companies is just one of many examples that result in health care by demand rather than need. Hyping marginal products and services in the private sector is standard practice. Health care should stop trying to emulate the private sector. The goal in health care is to conserve precious resources, not to create wealth for corporations as in the private sector.

- In a democratic free market society, consumers exercise freedom of choice in purchasing commodities. In the managed care concept of free markets, the citizen (employee) *is* the commodity and is auctioned off annually by his employer to the lowest bidder. The managed care market place where human beings are considered commodities is simply inconsistent with how a free market should operate in a democracy.

Managed Care Organizations and HMOs

One of the first items on the managed care agenda was to make physicians de facto employees. MCOs could then control both physicians' decision-making and reimbursement.

HMOs hired corporate attorneys to write contracts that contained financial incentives to limit care, gag clauses that prevented doctors from talking with patients about all of their therapeutic options, and "hold harmless clauses" that eliminated HMO liability for its policies as they affect the way physicians practice. Because of a poorly written law known as ERISA, MCOs were already shielded from legal action from patients harmed by their policies and actions. Physician contracts usually contained no fee schedules for services and procedures and often did not specify timeliness of payment. One might reasonably conclude that no one in his right mind would sign such a one-sided contract. But doctors did (usually without reading them). They had no choice. It was sign them or starve.

In addition, managed care plans used computer software to arbitrarily discount payments and bundle fees for separate procedures. They routinely rejected claims for trivial reasons stating that the claims weren't "clean"; they delayed payment by using such techniques as "losing" claims and by having multiple confusing addresses in the same area.

If all of the above weren't enough to put doctors at a disadvantage, there is a law that makes the playing field even less even. The McCarran Ferguson Act exempts insurance companies from federal antitrust scrutiny. Recall that the Goldfarb decision, cited above, removed antitrust exemption for physicians. So while MCOs can and do share all kinds of information including physician reimbursement schedules, physicians can be criminally prosecuted for sharing financial information as simple as office visit charges. These laws have prevented physicians from engaging in collective bargaining and allowed monopolistic insurance companies to dominate markets and force one-sided "take it or leave it" contracts upon physicians.

While clamping down on physician reimbursement,

highly profitable HMOs have seen fit to generously reward their management teams with enormous salaries and stock options. In 2001, corporate compensation for United Health Care CEO William McGuire was $54,129,501; the value of his unexercised stock options was a whopping $357,865,646. The compensation of William Taylor, retired chair of Cigna, was $24,741,578 with stock options worth $66,141,372. Space constraints prevent further listings.

In the past, MCOs have justified these outrageous salaries by pointing out how their organizations lowered overall health care costs. What is the value added by overpaid MCO executives now that health care costs are rising as sharply as they did before their arrival on the scene?

All the news is not bad, however; the tide is beginning to turn. Through legislation and the courts, organized medicine is leveling the playing field between MCOs and doctors. In the legislative arena, prompt pay bills have been enacted in most states. Class action suits against the large national MCOs have been filed. Early reports indicate that they will ultimately be successful. And when these suits are finally settled, the deceptive and dishonest practices of managed care will be a matter of public record. MCOs will pay massive financial penalties. More importantly, they will be forced to cease their egregious practices.

The Doctors

The centerpiece of managed care's effort to control costs was the "gatekeeper" primary care physician. The gatekeeper would approve or deny entry of all patients into the health care system. Primary care physicians were to be reimbursed under a system called capitation, which is a fixed monthly payment per patient. Physicians also would receive financial bonuses if they ordered fewer tests and procedures, and made fewer referrals to specialists. Fee-for-service payment was eliminated.

The gatekeeper concept is brilliant in theory, but, like all grandiose utopian schemes that depend on reforming human nature, it quickly broke down. First, no allowance was made for severity of illness in the panel of patients treated by a particular doctor. More importantly, physicians learned very quickly that HMOs rarely paid them their bonuses even if they practiced "economically." The HMOs kept the money and used it for shareholder profit and administrative salaries.

Doctors soon figured out that under gatekeeper HMOs, the way to maximize income was to forget about bonuses, have as many patients as possible on their panels, and spend as little time with them as possible. They began referring all patients with complex, time-consuming problems to specialists, even those patients whom they were qualified by training and experience to treat. This was the exact opposite of what the gatekeeper model was supposed to accomplish. Instead of the gate being closed, it was fixed in the open position. And, because the public had developed a mistrust of and antipathy toward HMOs, there wasn't a thing managed care could do to remedy this unanticipated and, from their standpoint, horrible turn of events.

Capitation, financial incentives and steeply discounted physician reimbursement have produced significant changes in the quality of care rendered by physicians. We now are hearing anecdotal reports about six-minute office exams and patients being examined without disrobing. Emergency room physicians often have to demand that sick Medicare HMO patients be admitted to the hospital over the objections of their primary care physicians, who assume financial risk and lose money when their patients are admitted. Inpatient Medicare HMO patients sometimes ask their hospitalists (physicians who care exclusively for hospitalized patients) if they are employed by insurance companies and will discharge them from the hospital too soon. Such questions indicate a loss of trust in the traditional doctor-patient relationship.

There is a crisis in overuse of emergency rooms; a problem that managed care boasted it would solve. In order not to examine sick, time-consuming patients, doctors' office telephone answering recordings say the following: "If you wish to see Dr. A, dial 1; for Dr. B, dial 2; for Dr. C, dial 3. If this is an emergency, call 911 and go to the nearest emergency room." Is it any wonder that emergency rooms are overcrowded? Any patient who thinks he or she has an urgent medical problem is advised to go to the emergency room.

Another way for physicians to extend the size of patient panels and increase revenue is to employ nurse practitioners. The original collaborative practice law where physicians work in conjunction with nurse practitioners was designed for medically underserved areas. The law was not intended to provide nurse practitioners for suburban areas where there is a plentiful supply of primary care physicians. Primary care physicians who believe that nurse practitioners are as well qualified to examine and evaluate patients as they are will someday find that they, themselves, are expendable and can be replaced by the very nurses that they have hired.

This same pressing need to see more patients in the office in order to generate more revenue explains the growth of hospitalists. Until recently, American doctors took care of their own hospitalized patients, calling in specialists when needed. But HMOs decided that physicians would not be compensated for seeing patients in the hospital. So, for financial reasons, doctors started referring patients to hospitalists. I do not intend to discuss here the pros and cons of hospitalists. But strictly from a cost analysis standpoint, it appears that hospitalists save little if any money. The MCO eliminates paying primary care physicians for hospital care but ends up paying hospitalists and the companies that employ them on a fee-for-service basis.

The growth of boutique medicine, where patients pay an annual fee from $1,000 to $5,000 just to obtain access to a physician who will spend enough time with them is a searing indictment of the assembly line kind of medicine practiced under managed care.

Capitation, reduced reimbursement, and the need to see large numbers of patients in short time intervals have failed to control costs, raised concerns about quality, and undermined the doctor-patient relationship.

The Patient

The public backlash against managed care came as a surprise to the industry. After all, for a mere $10 copayment, the patient could enter the health care system and practically everything else was "free." The managed care bureaucracy understood why physicians complained. They had, after all, taken away their authority and diminished their income. But the patients had a good deal. How could they be so ungrateful?

The public never articulated exactly what its problem with managed care was. Perhaps it was the moats and drawbridges it had to cross in getting authorizations for tests, procedures and consultations. Perhaps it was the high profile denials of care it read about in the media. Perhaps it was the lack of time the HMO doctors spent with the patients. Perhaps it was the lack of physician continuity and the way managed care treated the patient as a commodity like soybean futures or pork bellies to be auctioned off annually by their employer to the lowest HMO bidder. Perhaps it was a combination of all of these factors.

Spontaneous public expression of hostility toward HMOs reached unexpected heights in the 1997 movie "As Good As It Gets" starring Jack Nicholson and Helen Hunt. In the movie, Helen Hunt voices in strong terms her dissatisfaction with an HMO's treatment of her son's asthma and expresses her intention to obtain the services of a good independent non-HMO doctor. Unexpectedly, in movie houses all across the country, loud applause and cheering broke out after she spoke these lines. This spontaneous public reaction to "As Good As It Gets" was as bad as it gets for the HMO industry. Helen Hunt's comments will never be forgotten because they released a volcano of pent up public anger toward HMOs.

Public opinion can never be underestimated. No enterprise in a democratic society can survive very long without the support of public opinion—not a product, not a health care system, and not even a war. The managed care industry finally realized this. The best public relations firms' money could buy were unable to reverse the public's hostility to HMOs. As a result, the number of persons enrolled in HMOs is shrinking; the number enrolled in PPOs, a discounted fee-for-service system, is rising.

The Hospitals

Hospitals are the mirror image of managed care organizations. The same corporate CEOs who are responsible for managed care serve on hospital boards and thereby control hospitals. They remain committed to managed care, as do the administrators whom they hire. Hospitals like MCOs present the illusion that they are operating in a competitive free market and that they share the common goal of lowering health care costs. The facts indicate otherwise. Both are oligopolies; both are highly profitable.

The corporate CEOs who serve on the boards of academic medical centers also have compelled medical schools to accept managed care as the health care delivery system of the future and to incorporate its principles in their teaching curriculum. The CEOs hold the purse strings for endowed professorships, private research contributions, and the financial survivability of medical schools in general. It is not difficult to understand then why medical school deans and department chairs go along with the CEOs on managed care whether they like it or not.

The major mission of all hospitals is good patient care. But instead of focusing on that mission, hospitals have engaged in a variety of financially disastrous business ventures that have nothing to do with patient care. Most of these have been discussed at length previously in the series of articles on hospitals. They will be touched on briefly.

• *Horizontal mergers:* Hospitals proclaimed that savings would accrue from the formation of hospital networks due to economy of scale. There is no credible evidence to support this claim. Indeed studies show that independent

162 Arthur Gale MD

hospitals are just as efficient as networks. The major purpose of hospital mergers is to form oligopolies, which ultimately increase prices.

• *Vertical integration:* Hospitals told the public that the purpose of purchasing physician practices and owning HMOs was to improve efficiency. But financial losses have been staggering in the ownership of physician practices and HMOs. The real reason behind vertical integrations was to ensure referrals.

• *Colossal building projects:* One would never know that there is a fiscal crisis in health care from the way hospitals are building magnificent palaces that rival the finest luxury hotels. And when one hospital builds a palace, others copy its example. Capital improvements are necessary in any business, but current hospital construction is simply out of control.

All of the above activities are a waste of scarce resources. The taxpayer picks up much of the tab for this wasteful spending. The billions of dollars wasted on the above could be better spent on direct patient care and addressing such pressing problems as the nursing shortage.

And while we're mentioning the nursing shortage, allow me to digress briefly. Hospitals are begging the federal government to "do something" about the national nursing shortage. In my view, hospitals bear a major responsibility for the current nursing shortage. The cost-cutting measures of hospital "bean counters" is an attempt to "de-professionalize" nurses just like MCOs try to de-professionalize doctors. This has produced a crisis in morale causing many nurses to leave nursing. But the bean counters' actions have backfired. As a response to hospital cost-cutting measures that adversely affected patient care, nurses in California and elsewhere formed unions. The public and legislators got involved and now some state laws dictate nurse-patient ratios and other working conditions. The end result of interference in professional issues has counterproductively led to an actual increase in hospital costs.

Conclusion

The failure of so-called free market economics, as applied by managed care to control health care costs, disproves the theories of elitist policy makers in government, business, and academia, who sponsored managed care. It disproves the theories of the judges and antitrust lawyers at the FTC who scrapped Hippocratic ethics in the name of cost control. It disproves the theories of corporate CEOs who tried to remake health care in their own corporate image. And it disproves the theories of the managed care social engineers who thought that high health care costs were due to the fee-for-service system of payment that they would eliminate through capitation and financial incentives.

The take home lesson from the managed care experience is not to rely on so-called experts—the elitists who hold power in our society and who impose their views upon the citizens of our country without their approval. Thomas Jefferson said, "I know no safe depository of the ultimate powers of the society but the people themselves." In our democracy, and in a true market-driven economy, citizen consumers hold the power that ultimately will determine our future health care delivery system. When will our elected leaders and policy makers learn this lesson?